The Mother Year

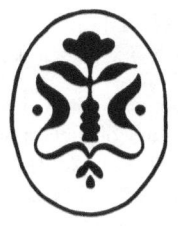

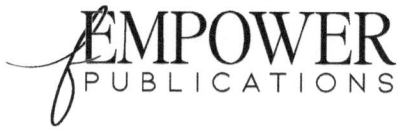

The Mother Year
Daily Reflections for the First Year of Motherhood
A Guide to Matrescence, The Transformative Journey of Becoming a Mother

fEMPOWER Press Trade Paperback Edition.
Copyright © 2025 Chelsey Scaffidi

Published in Canada, for Global Distribution
by fEMPOWER Publications
www.fempower.pub
For more information email: info@ygtmedia.co

ISBN trade paperback: 978-1-998721-11-5
ISBN hardback: 978-1-998721-01-6
eBook: 978-1-998754-93-9

To order additional copies of this book:
info@ygtmedia.co

The Mother Year

DAILY REFLECTIONS FOR THE FIRST YEAR OF MOTHERHOOD

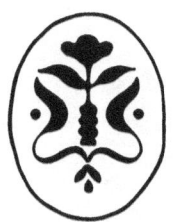

A GUIDE TO MATRESCENCE,
THE TRANSFORMATIVE JOURNEY OF BECOMING A MOTHER

CHELSEY SCAFFIDI

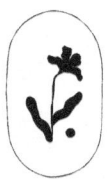

*To the mothers who, like me, felt the ground shift
beneath their feet in the initiation of motherhood and are,
with grace, finding their footing anew.*

*And to my January boys, Crusoe and Shiloh,
the catalysts of my rebirth. Like the snowdrop above,
you've shown me that the seasons of motherhood
are a sacred journey for us all.*

A woman's "Mother Year" is the first year her baby is earthside. This year-long recalibration, often felt as an initiation, is transformative, leaving no woman as it found her. Marking the beginning of motherhood, it entails a rebirth of a woman, from daughter to matriarch, from maiden to mother. In a word, this transition, the process of becoming a mother and the personal and physiological transformation that comes with it, is called *matrescence.*

Guide to The Mother Year

AUTUMN

Shedding the Maiden Self
MONTHS 1, 2, 3

WINTER

Becoming the Mother
MONTHS 4, 5, 6

SUMMER

The Mother's Bloom
MONTHS 10, 11, 12

SPRING

Seeds of the Mother
MONTHS 7, 8, 9

A Note on Pregnancy, A Preface of Sorts

There it was—a deep rose line against a field of white, gazing up at me like a silent herald. I stared at that pregnancy test for what felt like an eternity.

Motherhood had always been a distant constellation in my life's sky—a shimmering possibility without a mapped course, much like retirement: a future chapter to anticipate but not yet script. The years drifted by: college, law school, long days at a firm, and then finally landing my dream job as a lawyer in the nonprofit sector working on causes like climate change and human rights around the world. Life kept moving forward. My husband, always the practical one, had been ready to start a family for a few years.

So, when that dusky pink line appeared on a quiet Thursday morning, a whirlwind of emotions swept over me. There was awe . . . a profound sense of miracle that another life was unfolding within me—and there was trepidation . . . a weighty question echoing in my heart: Am I ready for this? I chose to keep the secret to myself, sharing it with no one, not even my husband. Not yet.

For the next three days, I went inward. I meditated, prayed, and tried to envision how this would all unfold. After what felt like the longest seventy-two hours of my life, I woke my husband at 6 a.m., suggesting we get an early, peaceful start to the day. Hand in hand, we wandered down to the docks, and that's when I told him what I already knew: We were having a baby.

He hugged me close. With tears in his eyes, he whispered, "We will do this together. You won't have to give up your dreams."

In that moment, I realized how much I needed his words without even knowing it. They made space for the parts of me still clinging to the life I loved. I feared losing myself—my ambitions, everything I'd worked so hard for up to that point. His reassurance gave me hope. Looking back, I wish I had known how much was about to change—how my dreams would completely transform, and how our lives were turning to one of the most beautiful chapters imaginable.

But first, my pregnancy would prove to be one of the hardest periods of my life.

In the weeks that followed the news, an unfamiliar fog settled over me, thick and unyielding. My body, which had once carried me effortlessly through each day, now felt foreign, exhausted by the smallest tasks. I had endless nausea with no cure but time, and a fatigue that ran deep to my bones. I could barely muster the energy to leave my bedroom. Where was the grounded, glass-half-full lawyer I knew that worked out daily and meditated regularly? She wasn't home.

My body demanded surrender—to soften, to yield. Then, at sixteen weeks, I woke up feeling okay. It was as if a magical spell had been lifted after being kissed by a frog (my husband would hate to be the frog here so let's keep that analogy between us). It was as if the curtains were lifted, and the sun could finally peek through.

Motherhood, I was learning, was an awakening. My pregnancy revealed two important lessons that have stuck with me.

First, mental health is fragile. Shifts in hormones and changes in the body are often out of our control and can quickly derail our thought patterns. In the deep spiritual transformation that comes with giving birth and becoming a mother, we are undoubtedly more vulnerable. Our hearts crack wide open as a baby and a mother are born. This transformation is known as matrescence—a term that encapsulates the complex physical, emotional, and social changes a woman undergoes when becoming a mother. Much like adolescence, matrescence is a period of significant growth and adaptation. Thus, I devoted myself to researching ways to support my mental stability in motherhood. I knew I couldn't control everything, but I wanted to do what I could. I encapsulated my placenta to help with the postpartum hormone drops, subscribed to eating an Ayurvedic meal plan for the first forty days after giving birth, and set gentle boundaries with friends and family to focus on healing. In short, I became deeply committed to cultivating practices and rituals to keep me rooted and connected to myself, ready to withstand the waves that motherhood brings—waves that can rise as tall as tsunamis.

Second, we are quick to forget. As I spoke openly about my first-trimester experience, I was shocked by how many of my friends and family nodded along because they, too, had had similar experiences in their pregnancy journey or knew someone who had. What? Why had no one ever mentioned that "morning sickness" lasts all day or that your food palette can completely change overnight? Perhaps it's by design—the quick forgetting that follows each stage, the blurring of pain and joy in the rearview mirror as we move forward. But I wanted to remember; I wanted to keep those raw, honest moments visible to capture the journey in all its complexity and growth. So, I wrote. And recorded. My plan was to even create a meditation centered around a theme for each day of my first year of motherhood. And then I had a baby. Therefore, my plan morphed into recording daily voice notes, writing partial journal entries, highlighting inspirational quotes in partially read pages of books, scribbling on sticky notes posted on my bathroom mirror—in short, it all became a collage of my experience, often with a few milk-stained pages. It wasn't polished, but it was real.

Those reflections are the heart of this book. I wanted to create something true—a companion to walk beside you in this first year of matrescence, the transition into becoming a mother. My hope is that this book adds a little sweetness to your days and a bit of softness to your journey; that it becomes a place where you can pause, take a breath, and find a sip of self-care when you need it most. May these pages hold space for you in quiet moments, offering comfort and understanding, whether you're wrapped in joy or wound up in struggle. May you find here the support I once sought—a reminder that you are not alone on this sacred path.

It's an honor to stand beside you. Truly.

Chelsey

The Mother Year

A POEM

If you had seen me that first year from the eye of a bird high above the clouds, my life may have appeared frozen, locked in place, caught against the backdrop of a swirling world.

Yet, I was always moving.

Moving from room to room, rocking, feeding, swaying, and tending to my baby. My movements were small, but purposeful, as I paced the floors of my home over and over. I spent more days in that space, or its orbit, than ever before. If you flew a bit closer, perched among the trees perhaps, my life may have looked somewhat recognizable.

Yet, everything was different.

Each day was a delicate dance of reorienting my new priorities with former commitments, reshaping my life's work up until this point. The lens through which I viewed the world had transformed, seemingly overnight. If you flew up to my windowsill now, peering in with curiosity, you may have even thought my physical form resembled what it once was.

Yet, a metamorphosis was unfolding within me.

I was shifting in ways unseen by the naked eye, slowly healing from birth. My organs, ribs, and womb were returning into place. My hormones were rearranging. My brain was making room for a new universe of thoughts, emotions, and instincts. My body may have seemed like mine once again but my nervous system and my heart would forever be intertwined with another being.

Yes, from the outside looking in, you might have missed these things.

But I felt it all.

My heart expanded. My soul stretched to embrace this new role. My divine assignment.

In truth, that year was one of profound transformation as I moved through the first year of my matrescence, the sacred process of *becoming* a mother.

This was ...
The Mother Year.

Introduction

I like to think of matrescence as the delicate, transformative dance of shape-shifting in motherhood. It's like a river that slowly carves a new path through the landscape of your soul, gently reshaping who you are. As you enter this sacred journey, you evolve, much like a flower opening to the sun's first light—you embrace new roles and emotions and bloom into a new version of yourself. It's a transition marked by the deepening of love, the awakening of nurturing instincts, the changing of the chemicals in your brain, and the morphing of the structure of your body; it is a profound realization that within you, a new life and a new self are tenderly growing together.

And so, it begins.

The first year of motherhood is different for everyone. It can be jolting, moving, beautiful, complicated, overwhelming, and overall, just a wild ride. Whatever it is, I can say with certainty that it will be different from what you expect. Because no book, podcast, or conversation can prepare you for the role you take on as you bring a new little being into this world and rebuild your life and yourself after your heart is cracked wide open. There are so many skills you learn by doing and so many feelings that bubble up on a moment's notice that trickle into your headspace when you least expect it.

I've heard the journey described this way: You are riding along a windy, tumultuous river in a wooden canoe with your baby. The undercurrent and weather are out of your control, so you must be alert and savvy in your navigation. Along the riverbanks stand the many people in your life. At their best, they offer wisdom, support, and love, but at their worst, they give unsolicited advice and judge. Ultimately, though, you are the one with the paddle in hand, and it's up to you to move forward with the best information you have. You will discover your own unique pathway in navigating these waters, but you have never taken this journey before; thus, it would be flippant to say simply to "trust your intuition" alone.

I believe our intuition is made of different parts, just like the body, and each part acts as a muscle that grows stronger when used. Your motherly intuition "muscle" began as a seed planted in pregnancy and continues to grow as you water it over time. You are learning a new skill set. You're recalibrating your existence and finding your footing as a woman reborn into motherhood. You are essentially going through the greatest initiation of your life on this river, and sometimes being the sole operator of the canoe means there is no one else to turn to when the waters get rough. And this can feel isolating, lonely even. In my hundreds of conversations with mothers in meditation circles, coffee walks, and interviews for this book, the word "lonely" was mentioned frequently. So, let's spend a moment with this concept.

Lonely is the feeling that comes from being "without others," whether a physical absence of other people (especially adults) to confide in or a lack of emotional/spiritual support you can connect with on a deeper level. It is, in essence, when you look around and recognize there is no one else in the canoe with you other than your sweet baby.

In contrast, the feeling of being *alone*, however, means to be "with Self." For some of us, motherhood is one of the first times in our lives when we spend long stretches of time with Self, especially in the early months when so much is required of us. For some women, the feeling of being alone is a welcome reprieve from the social swirlings of their pre-baby life. For others, this new reality may feel like being in a foreign land they never intended to visit.

Here is where this book comes in.

During my own Mother Year, I sometimes felt lonely (without others on my same journey), then found it challenging to embrace the sacred sweetness of being alone (with myself) during other moments. So, I journaled, recorded voice notes, scratched down little poems about my experience, and most importantly, tried to capture the words I needed to hear that day to paddle on. At the end of the year, I listened to my recordings and cried many times when hearing the crack of my voice, the raw feelings and honest dialogue flowing from my heart straight out of my lips. Those recordings are now memorialized in this book. The pages that follow are little messages in a bottle I have sent down the river for you to find at the right moment in your (very) few moments of stillness each day. Some are written as reflections of the days past, and some are recorded from a moment of time. Either way, I hope these words feel nourishing, energizing, and like a hug from a good friend. Imagine me as your fellow paddler as you read the words of another mother on the *exact day* you are in now.

When you hold this book, remember that there are others around you, all over the world. There are mothers rowing behind you (with a baby younger than yours), in front of you (with a baby older than yours), and even alongside you (in a similar timeline of your motherhood journey). In addition to sifting back through my own notes while writing this book, I also interviewed one hundred women about their Mother Year journey. The names of those women are lovingly printed in the back of this book, and their energy is infused within these pages. Each time you open this book, I invite you to feel the power of those women, the women who shared their hardest moments and longest days, the women who are with you, silently cheering you on from afar, no matter where they float on the river. Place your hand on your heart and receive that energy and support from the collective.

And if you take away nothing else, Mama, remember this:

You matter. You deserve to be seen, held, and "mothered" in the most loving way.

You are so powerful.

And you are doing a good job.

WHAT IS THIS BOOK?

The Mother Year is a daily resource of uplifting and honest messages for your first year of motherhood. It's not to say that the other years that follow this first one aren't important, but there's something particularly potent, jarring, and special about the first trip around the sun as you transition from "daughter" or maiden into your full expression as "mother." Think of this book as a friend walking beside you as you move through this profound initiation of *becoming*. Starting on the day your baby is born (Day 1), I invite you to use these pages as a daily act of self-love, nourishment, and rebellion against the preconceived notions you were likely told about this year and how you would feel. There is so much outside of our control, but one thing within our power is how we nurture our own sense of self, both as a woman and as a mother.

Each daily entry includes a prayer, something I found deeply meaningful in my own journey. As a Christian, my prayers reflect my faith, and my hope is that they help you connect with God. Though rooted in my beliefs, I trust these prayers will offer comfort and guidance no matter where you are on your spiritual path. My intention is for them to bring you peace and support as you navigate the beautiful chaos of motherhood. May they be a source of strength and help you feel God's loving presence as you walk your own path.

You've likely encountered a barrage of advice and opinions from the moment your pregnancy began, advice often centered around feeding, diapers, sleeping, or other *practical* aspects of childcare. I'm not interested in any of that. This book is not meant to be an instruction guide on how to care for your baby; instead, it's about how to care for yourself. Even without knowing you personally, I trust that you are the best mother for your baby. Your intuition is your greatest gift. This book is about navigating the internal themes that might arise during your Mother Year, not a judgment or a prescribed model for your external environment. I only share specific stories to illustrate the reality of certain days and how I worked through those situations to tend to my own transformation. There are hundreds of other books that discuss schedules, nutrition, products, and so on. This book is solely about nourishing your *soul*, Mama. And nothing else.

On a related note, while I share insights rooted in my own experience with biological birth and the mother–child bond, I deeply recognize and honor the many other paths to motherhood, including surrogacy and adoption. Each journey is unique, and I aim for this book to speak to all who embrace the beautiful transformation of becoming a mother.

HOW TO USE THIS BOOK:

The Mother Year is divided into four parts that I affectionately refer to as "seasons." As mothers, we tend to view our journey in distinct phases (think of the term "trimesters" in pregnancy), and I've found that significant shifts in perspective often occur about every three months during a woman's Mother Year. You'll begin in the *Autumn* season for months one to three, followed by *Winter* in months four to six, *Spring* in months seven to nine, and finally, *Summer* in months ten to twelve. Each season opens with a scannable QR code that links to meditations for that particular time of your Mother Year.

Throughout this book, you'll also find short practices sprinkled in, called *Sips of Self-Care*. As a mother, it's vital to pour back into yourself, even in small, intentional ways. These micro moments are designed to fit seamlessly into your motherhood journey, requiring less than five minutes each. Their purpose is simple: to create gentle pauses that refresh your heart and leave you feeling grounded, rejuvenated, and inspired.

These practices are not rooted in traditional ideas of self-care, which often suggest indulgent or time-consuming rituals. Instead, I view self-care as a way of replenishing your inner reserves—restoring the balance and vitality you need to show up fully in your life. The *Sips of Self-Care* in this book embody this philosophy. These small but meaningful pauses are invitations to refill your cup, one mindful moment at a time.

Some days will present challenges, but every day will present some aspect of joy and growth. Within these moments lie the beautiful and inspiring experiences that make this journey worthwhile.

So, let's navigate your *Mother Year* together, Mama, day by day.

Please note that if you don't know the exact day of motherhood you are on, you can search "how many days since [insert baby's birthdate]" on the internet and it will show you the number so you can follow along with the daily references.

(*Autumn*)

SHEDDING THE MAIDEN SELF

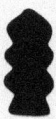

THE FIRST QUARTER:

RELEASING, UNRAVELING, WELCOMING

"It's only when we are cracked open that the light can begin to seep in."

*Scan for meditations to guide you
through this season*

Autumn: Shedding the Maiden Self
RELEASING . UNRAVELING . WELCOMING

This first season of the Mother Year is Autumn.

Picture this scene in your mind's eye: The canopy of leaves is transforming from hues of green to yellow, orange to red, and finally to brown before gently dropping from the towering oak tree. We begin here because, for us, too, this marks a season of separation, a separation from the version of yourself that existed before you cradled this tiny being in your arms, before you felt the beauty, weight, and heart-swelling responsibility of being someone's home. In this season, you're falling deeply in love with your baby, and as you move toward this love, you unconsciously move *away* from something else. That "something else" is the external world, the social web you once spun, and the culture that whispers the falsehood in your ear that your worth stems from what you produce rather than who you are.

Continuing with our nature analogy, I like to think of these early months as the "newborn forest," a place where the overwhelming growth of new life envelops you like a dense, uncharted wilderness. Much like wandering in a thick forest, you find yourself in a world where each day is shaped by the needs of your newborn, and it's difficult to see the bigger picture or to look beyond the immediate moment. It's a time of navigation and feeling your way through the undergrowth, where the terrain is still too dense to fully understand or appreciate the broader landscape of your life. Time within our home seems to meld together: phone calls go unanswered, messages remain unread, and emails? Let's just say they, too, start piling up.

You, Mama, are *in it*. Your cup is brimming emotionally and physically. During this season, there's scarcely any energy left for what lies beyond you and your baby.

This process of becoming a mother transforms every woman it touches. Matrescence educator, Nikki McCahon, describes it this way: "it unravels her and rebuilds her. It cracks her open, takes her to her edges. It's both beautiful and brutal, often at the same time."[1] This initial season, dear Mama, is the unraveling. And while "unraveling" might seem to imply coming apart, its true gift lies in *opening* what is tightly held, in allowing the tangled places to ease, in welcoming what is ready to emerge. In this gentle undoing, the mystery of motherhood stretches before you—not to be solved, but to be lived. Each loosened thread is an invitation to weave yourself anew. Let this unfolding be the beginning of a beautiful remaking.

While we're labeled "mothers" from the moment our babies are born, the truth is that this transition involves a profound spiritual initiation, one that's both breathtakingly beautiful and unrelentingly challenging. This initiation necessitates a profound sacrifice as we navigate this uncharted territory.

As women, stepping into motherhood is one of the most profound shifts of our lives. It's so significant that a term has been coined for it: matrescence (pronounced muh-tres-sense). Matrescence encompasses the physical, emotional, hormonal, and social shift into motherhood. Yes, our brains literally change, as do our bodies, perspectives, priorities, and so much more. We've given birth to our babies, but we're also giving birth to ourselves.

Think again of those leaves on the oak tree—let them be your inspiration during this season. They don't struggle to hold on; they let go, understanding that this is all part of the journey and knowing that eventually, they'll return brighter and stronger, following the cues of nature.

So, in this season, I offer these words to cradle and guide you:

- Be assured that this time is sacred and temporary.
- Embrace the space between you and the outer world.
- Activate your faith over your fears.
- Calm your mind and open your heart.
- Surrender with grace.
- Remember, you possess more strength than you realize.

You've got this, Mama.

I am a mother

You did it, beautiful Mama. Whatever your birth story entails, here you are. Forever changed, and probably in utter disbelief over just how quickly your life, and everything in it, can take on a different hue. I'll keep this brief because, honestly, words fall short during this period of immense emotion. We often get swept up in the adrenaline of this time, so I invite you to *slow down* and find gratitude for the life you've created and nurtured within your body. Your care and strength are the reasons why this being has entered the world today. And you should feel so proud.

(A PRAYER FOR TODAY)

God, thank you for blessing me with this new little human.
I stand in awe of the miracle that is life.

Still in the primal element

You've experienced something miraculous. You've brought life into being. At this moment, the elemental drive to love, provide for, and safeguard your baby is so palpable because your baby is an extension of you. It's the first time you've ever had another part of yourself on the earth—distinct in the physical realm yet deeply interconnected emotionally and spiritually. What you're feeling is novel, which can be unsettling and, in some ways, even frightening. This is a period of change, adjustment, and reorientation.

It's also okay to be in complete shock and awe of this new role you're embodying.

(A PRAYER FOR TODAY)

God, help me remember that I was chosen to be this child's mother, and my purpose, my place, and my power are right here.

Celebrate your evolution

Are you feeling like a caterpillar? Mother and baby cocooned together, wrapped in a world of tenderness and new beginnings? You are entering a deep metamorphosis. You are changing from inside out, at a cellular level. Everything is evolving.

Although the analogy of the cocoon stage is often considered the beginning of the butterfly's story, the tale, much like yours today, began much earlier. It started with a tiny egg, carefully placed on a leaf by the mother butterfly. This egg, no larger than a pinhead, then hatches, and a small caterpillar emerges. Over the next period, the caterpillar has an innate desire to grow, an insatiable hunger to nourish itself on every level. It consumes large numbers of leaves, shedding its skin multiple times as it outgrows its current form—something you experienced throughout your many chapters of pregnancy. Despite its small size, the caterpillar is remarkably efficient, transforming the food it eats into body mass, preparing for significant changes ahead. As the caterpillar reaches its full size, it becomes less focused on nourishment and more on finding a safe place to begin its next transformation, its rebirth. Here, it sheds its final larval skin and enters the pupal stage, where the magic of metamorphosis truly begins.

You are here. You grew your baby within your body and expanded your heart and mind in every way. Here, you stand on the precipice of this next chapter with transformation at your feet. Celebrate how far you've come. Celebrate your growth and evolution. Celebrate your initiation into motherhood. You deserve to be celebrated at every stage, Mama.

(A PRAYER FOR TODAY)

God, thank you for this gift. Thank you for my body. Thank you for my creativity. Thank you for my soul. Thank you for this beautiful evolution.

Seeing the world as a mother

I was living in Chicago when my son was born. It was cold outside, but the warmth I felt inside the walls of our home was tangible. We lit candles, played records, and switched between various calming Spotify playlists. In retrospect, this time holds some of my favorite moments because we kept it so sacred. We ordered in food and kept our number of visitors to a minimum.

Inside my body, I felt warmth too. As I looked out my window, I saw my neighbor's children playing in the leaves, piling them together and giggling as they rolled in the various colors of shredded debris from the trees. I had lived in this house for years and had seen these kids before, but it hadn't struck me the same way. Someone had raised these children; someone was their *mother.*

I also sensed a difference when I turned on the TV. I selected a series I had been watching the week prior to giving birth, but somehow, in that moment, the sounds, colors, and even the language of the show felt overwhelming. Not much time had passed, but my perspective on the world had changed; my heart was wide open.

I turned off the TV, put on my favorite song, and prepared myself a cup of tea. These, at least I could be sure, provided a safe haven.

(A PRAYER FOR TODAY)

God, thank you for softening my gaze and opening my eyes in this role of motherhood. Transform me into someone who understands that everything happens for my highest good and allow me to love the parts of myself that are evolving in motherhood.

Sip of Self-Care:

Safeguard yourself by being mindful of what you expose your eyes, ears, and mind to during this early postpartum period. See if you can approach your responses to certain people, media, or situations with curiosity, and use this as a guide to decipher who/what should or should not be in your bubble of peace.

Adrenaline to the heart

New motherhood can be an exhilarating rush. Overwhelmingly tired and overstimulated, my body is still recalibrating, still healing (oh, so much healing to come). I strive to maintain faith in myself, yet I find myself oscillating between living in a dream cloud, questioning whether it's all real, and being overwhelmed by the constant need to be "on it" while learning as I go.

This all prompts a rush of cortisol in our brains and bodies. Some view cortisol as the stress hormone, but stress and excitement elicit similar responses. You may be experiencing a bit of both right now. Perhaps you're forgetting to eat; you're likely awake at all hours. How DO you manage everything? What fuels this newfound energy? I believe it's this feeling, this sensation that nothing can prepare you for. It's as if your heart is entirely exposed, wide open to the world, filled with an intense sense of love, and so much so that it's challenging to remember (or imagine) life before this tiny person was part of it. Amid the adrenaline coursing through my body, I realize it's pooling in my heart, fueling me to carry on.

(A PRAYER FOR TODAY)

God, I'm grateful for the breath in my lungs and the blessings around me. You've designed me to sustain life not only for my baby but also for myself. Today, help me remember what a miracle I am, and may I feel ease and peace within my heart and mind.

Rest + Recharge, Here + Now

Don't be misled into thinking that this time, right here and now, serves any purpose other than resting, resetting, and recalibrating for you. These moments are the embers of your motherhood. Tend to the flame—feed it, let it breathe, protect it. Your world is meant to slow down during this period.

Friends and loved ones are eager to see the baby and catch up with you, but they'll still be there when you're ready. I recognize that it's not always easy to set those boundaries. As a recovering lifelong people pleaser, I would have felt more challenged in this department had it not been for the COVID pandemic that required us to have a limited number of visitors. Allow this time to envelop you like a secret cocoon. You don't need to let anyone in until you feel it's time.

This is a truly special, fleeting period. Absorb every last drop of it.

(A PRAYER FOR TODAY)

God, I'm grateful for the energy that has fueled me these past few days. Help me recognize that I'm also deserving of care. May I find substantial pockets of rest, and may my body heal with peace and tranquility.

The remnants of your birth

Whether your birthing experience was smooth or turbulent, it transforms you. It opens your body, mind, and spirit in ways you never imagined. Your nervous system wonders what happened. Remember that processing this monumental event takes time.

I find myself experiencing flashbacks—little snippets of a movie playing in my mind when the house is still and quiet. It's a common question for people to ask about your birth story, and with each retelling, you may find that new details emerge, painting a fuller picture of what transpired. You have plenty of time to process, celebrate, and heal. For now, let the remnants of your birthing experience flow through you as you digest the enormity of what you underwent just one week ago. Begin to meditate on what you may need to heal from or metabolize from the experience.

(A PRAYER FOR TODAY)

God, thank you for the strength and power to cross the threshold of birth. Today, as I find gratitude for any part of the experience that brought me joy, may any heaviness from the gravity of birth begin to dissipate.

Birth is just the beginning

During pregnancy, the idea of giving birth feels like the finish line. We count down the days until baby is here. We spend months preparing ourselves, our minds, our partners, and our spaces. We read books, do research, and talk to other mama friends. However, as I crossed that threshold and welcomed my son into this world, I realized that while birth marked the end of one chapter, it also marked the beginning of a new one. It was as if, after reaching the "finish line," I immediately returned to the race. But this time, I didn't have nine months to plan; I learned by doing, seeing, and responding. It was all overwhelming for me—the realization there was no clear endpoint on this path, that this was a permanent state change, the role of motherhood, etc. Here is what helped me: instead of viewing this journey as a series of milestones on a long road, what if we see it as a leisurely walk? As an opportunity to get curious, to notice the changing color of the canopy of leaves that adorn our lives? As time to note the subtle shifts from season to season in our hearts?

(A PRAYER FOR TODAY)

God, grant me strength on the days I feel unprepared or unsure. Let signs and subtle reminders from my angels above guide me.

Sip of Self-Care:

Close your eyes and imagine walking through a stone-walled doorway into an unfamiliar garden. Breathe and let your mind wander for several minutes, envisioning how this new terrain looks for you. Whisper to yourself, "I am a mother." Notice how that sentence reverberates through your being.

Your mama intuition begins as a seed—give it time to grow

Tonight, the smallest decision triggered my doubt. My partner and I debated where to put our baby to sleep: in bed with us or in the bassinet. I made a choice, then second-guessed it. I laid there awake, questioning my decision. Finally, after a few deep breaths, my husband whispered, "What's wrong?" I confessed I wanted to change my initial decision. Given that it had taken almost an hour to put our baby to sleep, my partner was hesitant.

As soon as we attempted to move him, my son woke up, screaming. I crumbled. Had I made the wrong choice? Was my initial decision "right"? I felt torn and tired, and on top of it, I had a crying little one who now needed twenty more minutes of bouncing to fall back asleep. There was even a hint of shame. Here I was, his mother, and I didn't know the right answer.

The truth is, our maternal intuition and savviness to navigate this new path grows stronger *over time*. There's immense pressure and countless decisions to be made during those early days. We, as mothers, are learning too.

Remember that just as your baby is new to the world you, too, are learning, and that's okay. Second-guessing decisions while finding your footing is perfectly normal.

(A PRAYER FOR TODAY)

God, bless me with peace, confidence, and self-assurance. Help me find moments of stillness amid chaos, allowing my spirit to rest and recharge. Surround me with a supportive community offering guidance, love, and understanding.

Piecing yourself back together

One of the most surprising realizations after giving birth is the time it takes to heal. Did you know (I certainly didn't) that it takes over five weeks after birth for the uterus to return to its pre-pregnancy size—usually around forty days? From soreness and aches to bleeding and other postpartum ailments, healing simply requires rest. Additionally, like most healing in life, postpartum recovery isn't linear—it involves profound emotional, mental, and physical restoration. Be gentle today. Do less than you think you can. Even if your physical healing progresses, remember that your internal healing needs time too. Just as autumn prepares for winter, this chapter of early motherhood prepares you for the lifetime ahead, so give yourself the space to find solid ground for you and your baby.

(A PRAYER FOR TODAY)

God, transform me into someone who always recognizes and respects my inner worth. Guide me to the right actions at the right time in this wobbly period.

A lifetime of learning

It's been less than two weeks, but it feels like my entire world has changed. Maybe you feel the same way. Some moments, I feel like I've figured it out, and then the next moment, my baby develops something called cradle cap and I'm back to researching. I wonder if this feeling of "always something new just around the riverbend" will ever cease. Deep down, I know the answer is no. Our babies will constantly change, which means we, as mothers, will too. We'll always be learning along the way.

But on Day 11, when my sisters visited, something profound happened. They wanted to hold the "little squishy baby." I went to shower, and as I stepped into the warm water, my whole body relaxed. Later, one sister entered the bathroom and asked questions, and I realized then that I knew a lot about my baby: his communication cues, his favorite sleeping position, and how he likes to be soothed. He is my world, and I am his. In less than two weeks, I already know all that.

Wow, I thought, *I'm pretty amazing.*

And so are you, Mama.

(A PRAYER FOR TODAY)

God, in moments of doubt, help me understand my worth in your eyes. Guide me to see myself as you see me—loved, cherished, and infinitely valued.

A new normal

I am amazed by how quickly this current routine has become my new normal. I can't even remember the days before I was calculating the time between feeds or napping with a little warm body next to mine. I honestly can't recall when my hips didn't instinctively sway or when I wasn't on the lookout for diaper rash. Those days when I wore regular bras (without milk stains) or had a charged phone (and could find my phone, for that matter) seem like clouds of dust in the rearview mirror. And it's not good or bad, it's just what is. Life is more rewarding and fulfilling when we can *really be* in the moment before us.

What he looks like, smells like, and the way his hands curl instinctively into a ball—when we allow what is in front of us to be *the* interesting things we are excited for (as opposed to waiting in anticipation for what's next), life becomes more vibrant, full, and overall, just more enjoyable.

People have begun stopping me on the street to say things like "I remember when my son/daughter was that little. Enjoy this period." I can feel that they mean it, from the nostalgia and the hint of sadness in their tone. I know I will miss this chapter, when my little one is so small.

Therefore, I want to soak it all in. Every inch. While I can.

(A PRAYER FOR TODAY)

God, may I feel peace knowing I am exactly where you called me to be in this moment.

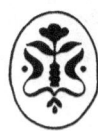

Sip of Self-Care:

Make a mental note of two things that have changed since your baby was born. How have you changed? Your priorities? Your schedule? Notice any emotions or feelings that arise as you think about these changes. Put one hand on your heart, one hand on your belly. Whisper the following words as you close your eyes and breathe:

"I welcome this new version of me."

"I honor this sacred time in my life."

The gateway

The early days of motherhood are often referred to as "the gateway" because they mark the profound and transformative beginning of a lifelong journey. Just as a gateway serves as an entrance to a new realm, the birth of a child opens up a world of boundless love, joy, and responsibility for a mother. It's a period of intense adjustment, learning, and self-discovery as a woman steps into the role of mother, navigating the challenges and joys of caring for her newborn. The term "gateway" symbolizes the transition into this pivotal phase of life; it's filled with the promise of growth and the forging of an unbreakable, lifelong bond between a mother and her child.

In the gateway, you may feel a flurry of emotions as fears and thoughts move through you. In fact, according to Chinese postpartum tradition collectively referred to as *zuo yue zi* (the "sitting month"), giving birth is one of the three moments in a woman's life when she is both most open as well as experiencing changes and is therefore susceptible to physical and emotional strain.[2] With so many moving parts in this period, it's important to slow down, rest, and limit outside distractions and movement (to the extent you can). Let this period be one of healing. Let this be a time when you send down new roots to reground yourself from the whirlwind of birth.

(A PRAYER FOR TODAY)

God, fill me with a sense of awe and wonder for this transformational period. Grant me the strength and courage to navigate these changes with grace, and may your restorative love bring peace and renewal to my body, mind, and spirit.

Honor your birth alongside theirs

For you, this is a sacred journey, a profound rite of passage that touches the very essence of your soul. In this moment, your spirit reconnects with its primal essence, reborn through the transformative power of motherhood. You stand at the threshold of a new realm, embodying divinity itself.

For your baby, their birth is a profound awakening. They emerge from the cocoon of their your womb—a sanctuary of gentle rhythms and soothing warmth. As they enter the world, it's as if they're waking up from a serene dream into a vibrant, dazzling expanse of light and sound. The comforting embrace they once knew is replaced by crisp, cold air and a lively kaleidoscope of voices and faces. The transition from the familiar fluid haven to this new, sensory-rich world is likely both wondrous for them and overwhelming—a shift from a cherished bubble to a bright, slightly disorienting reality.

Honor this sacred rebirth for both you and your baby. Embrace the emotions that arise, let tears flow freely, laugh with abandon, and find profound peace within yourself as you nurture both your own spirit and the precious new life you hold.

(A PRAYER FOR TODAY)

Guide me to honor the rebirth of my soul.

You are allowed to F E E L

During these first few weeks, you may be buzzing from all the "firsts" and the newness of it all. You are learning how to do everything from diaper changes to feeding on demand to the dozen other actions that are required of you as a mother. It's easy to fall into the role of "doing" as we step into caring so intently for another human being while also trying to tend to the basic needs of ourselves (hello, wonderful five-minute shower). But underneath the waves of the day, there are so many hormones swirling through our postpartum bodies. I recall sitting in the rocking chair for a moment while my husband was downstairs changing our baby, and in the stillness, this moment to myself, all I really wanted to do was cry. So, I did. And it felt *so incredibly good*. It wasn't a cute cry—it was cathartic. It was a release. And it was needed.

Let this entry today be a reminder to you that you are allowed to feel it all. Our emotions are simply energy in motion, and the more we try to push them down and away, the longer they stay trapped within us. When we let ourselves experience the emotion rising within, we can move freely through it. Our emotions can rise and dissipate faster and with more ease.

So, cry if you need to cry.

Let it all out. Your feelings are valid and by tending to them, you show self-love to the woman woven within the mother—you.

(A PRAYER FOR TODAY)

Today, let me remember that I am a vessel for my emotions, a safe passage for them to move through. May I hold myself with compassion as I welcome each feeling into the sanctuary of my heart.

Unclench your fingers

Before our babies come into the world, we plan a lot. We decorate the nursery and make checklists of the items we "think" we need. But after they arrive? The plans go out the window. In these first few weeks, I often found myself holding on to the way I thought things should be instead of listening to my intuition. On this particular day, I was trying to use a trending swaddle I bought for my son, but he didn't like it. It was a lovely fabric and the sweetest color. It didn't matter. He loathed it.

Finally, after several failed attempts and tough moments for both of us, I surrendered. My husband went out to the nearest store and bought another one (not nearly as cute, I might add), but it worked. When I put him in it, he settled right down. As I laid there, gazing at this sleeping angel in his new sleep sack, I heaved a sigh of relief. It felt good to let go. There is always resistance before release, and this was a lesson I needed to learn. My expectations and plans can be helpful, sure, but a looser grip on the outcome is better for everyone, including myself.

(A PRAYER FOR TODAY)

God, help me release the grip of control that I sometimes hold too tightly. Grant me the courage to trust your plan and belief in my abilities. Fill my heart with peace as I embrace the journey of letting go, finding comfort in the knowledge that you are guiding every step I take.

Sip of Self-Care:

Clench your fists tightly, scrunch your toes, close your eyes and breathe in—hold for a count of three. Now open your eyes and let your breath out, releasing all the tension in your body, unfurling your fingers and toes. Notice the amount of effort it takes to be rigid and hold tight versus the feeling of softening, opening, and allowing.

My favorite love story is ours

Whether it was love at first sight for you and your baby or whether it took some time after birth, you are co-creating a love story of a lifetime with the sweet soul in your arms. Isn't it interesting that we use the term "falling in love" when describing the deepest of human connections. Because the act of falling is an act of *surrender*. For it's in the risk, the vulnerability, and the trust required to let down our guard that we let ourselves love another human in such a way. What an act of faith . . . to soften, to release our walls and allow love to reach the deepest parts of our soul. If we are closed off, love couldn't permeate our heart space the way it does in motherhood. What a truly magnificent thing you have done, Mama. What a beautiful love story you are unfolding.

(A PRAYER FOR TODAY)

God, thank you, thank you, thank you for bringing me the greatest love I have ever known.

Rebalance your energy centers

In Ayurveda (one of the world's oldest whole-body healing systems), there are three categories of energy called "doshas" that exist in all of nature, including us. They are Vata (air), Pitta (fire), and Kapha (earth).

Following pregnancy and birth, mothers are believed to have excess Vata energy because their bodies contain light, air, dry, and cold qualities resulting from the spiritual opening of becoming a mother, the physical loss of energy, blood, and fluids from their bodies during birth, and the liminal space that exists in the belly where their newborn once lived. Additionally, they are sleep-deprived and experiencing a high level of adrenal fatigue in tending to their babies, further adding to the Vata imbalance, which rules the nervous system.

Therefore, incorporating nourishment and self-care practices that have warm, smooth, oily, and stable qualities are recommended for at least the first forty days postpartum. Try to eat only warm foods with grounding spices like turmeric and ginger. Avoid cold or dry foods as they further deplete your Vata energy. Try leaving your morning smoothie for twenty minutes until it's room temperature or drinking bone broth throughout the day. Hot baths and self-massage are also wonderful options for bringing in earth energy to combat the Vata imbalance and calm the nervous system (I recommend using Ashwagandha Bala oil each day).

There are many recipes and practices available to harness the power of foods, herbs, and massage to support those qualities you want. These small changes can make a tremendous impact on the way you feel in this postpartum period.

(A PRAYER FOR TODAY)

Help me remember that my body is a vessel and a temple and what I put in it and around it is important. Allow the healing energy of these foods and practices to bring me comfort and balance, leaving me feeling more connected to you, God.

The power of "and"

Lately, I have been asked many times, "How are you doing?" Honestly? I'm not sure, and it's not because I've lost touch with my feelings but because I'm feeling so many things *all at once*. It's like trying to paint a picture of my life but not knowing which color to choose.

This morning in my meditation, the session centered around the power of "and," and it felt like the key that unlocked my voice. This is so central to mindset reframes, because when connected to a really hard thought or uncomfortable feeling, using the word "and" has the power of connecting us to that which is going well, which directs us upward instead of into a downward spiral.

The truth is, as mothers, we often experience two or more (often conflicting) feelings simultaneously, or side by side, and this serves as the basis for human consciousness—the ability to hold more than one feeling at once. What I've come to realize is that these feelings are all ingredients that make our journey into motherhood unique.

No one has quite the same recipe.

So, when people ask me this question now, I answer authentically. I say things like "I am utterly exhausted *and* enamored with my baby" or "It's the hardest thing I've ever done *and* I'm taking it day by day." This feels true and complete. These feelings, experiences, and sensations come together like the beautiful fall leaves on a big oak tree. The variety of colors are breathtaking. Let it all be okay. Let it all be seen.

(A PRAYER FOR TODAY)

Today and every day, may I remember there is power in the pause, power in the "and." That life is ours for co-creating with you, God. In the swirl of emotions that motherhood brings, help me embrace the intricate blend of feelings, knowing that they shape my journey with authenticity and depth.

The dance

Think back to when you first met your partner, or your best friend. In those interactions, was it smooth? Was the connection and "knowing of one another" instant? Did it always feel easy? For my husband and me, there was a period of doing what I like to call "the dance." He would text, then I would analyze his words, wondering what he *really* meant before I responded. We would meet, and it would take a few minutes of smirking and light chatter before delving into the deeper conversation. As time went on, however, we got more comfortable reading each other's mannerisms, body language, and tone of voice. The more familiar we became with one another, the easier it was to find our rhythm.

This pattern repeats itself in most human relationships, and the one with you and your baby is no different. However, when your dance partner is a newborn (who has a completely different communication style), it can feel a little bumpy before the rhythm starts to really settle in. You are doing so much, often for the first time, and you are likely sleep-deprived and physically tired from the repetitive demands of this initial period. Emotions are high and the decisions feel endless, but I promise you, you and your baby will find *your unique rhythm.*

Let this period be one where you give yourself grace as you find your footing. You learn by doing, so let the dance, the starts and stops, the changing rhythm be okay as you build the relationship between you and your baby.

(A PRAYER FOR TODAY)

God, give me the strength and wisdom to navigate this new journey of motherhood. Help me find the patience to soothe the tears, the understanding to decode the cries, and the tenderness to provide comfort. Guide my hands and heart as I care for this little one.

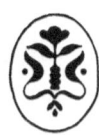

Sip of Self-Care:

The "dance" likely has you paying attention to feeding schedules, diaper changes, and the sleep patterns of your baby. But today, I invite you to really pay attention to your input as much as your output. Are you eating nutritious foods? Are you staying hydrated? As the lead, it is so incredibly important that you feel taken care of on an emotional, physical, and psychological level.

Embrace the dawn

The days with your new baby often may feel more manageable than the nights because daylight aligns with our natural rhythms. Your little one may still be catching up on sleep during the day while their circadian rhythm settles. Yet the nights can stretch long and lonely, with diaper changes and feedings breaking your rest. In these moments, remember that each night always gives way to morning eventually, offering a fresh start.

Motherhood brings our inner shadows into sharp focus. It's a journey filled with both breathtaking beauty and challenging terrain. Some days are serene and picturesque, while others feel like a battleground of thoughts. In every moment, seek the light. If you find yourself struggling, don't hide from it—acknowledge and accept it. Reach out to a friend or seek support. Remember, this phase is temporary, and knowing you're not alone brings a profound sense of peace.

Even the darkest night yields to the dawn. As the world turns, know that the sun *will return to you*, physically and metaphorically. When morning arrives, take a deep breath, open the blinds, and welcome the light.

(A PRAYER FOR TODAY)

God, in the middle of the long nights, send me a sense of peace and a reminder that I am not alone. You are always with me, as are mothers around the world who are loving and tending to their babies. Give me the peace that is felt in your presence and the presence of others.

Motherhood as an ocean

Motherhood is like the ocean in that it encompasses a depth of emotions and experiences that are vast and profound. Just like the ocean's currents and tides shape the landscape around it, the journey of motherhood is continuously carving up and softening the structures *within us—our heart, intuition, mind, and soul.* The shaping is constant; it's slowly leaving its mark on who we are as a woman, partner, and friend. And as beautiful as the ocean is, it is also unpredictable. Sometimes we can see above the waves to feel the sun on our faces, and in other moments, we may feel swept away in its turbulent tides. In some moments, we are faced with mild conditions, and by the next hour, the thrashing waves are upon us.

But when we start to see the vastness that motherhood is, we can connect to the grounded mother energy *below* the waves that is not as susceptible to the surface conditions. Below the waves is a sense of calm, peace, and understanding. The more we connect to the stability within us, the easier it is to ride the current of conditions that present themselves in our day-to-day lives.

(A PRAYER FOR TODAY)

Dear God, in the midst of so much change, I ask for your unwavering presence. Grant me the strength to endure, the wisdom to navigate, and the patience to await the clearing skies above. With you by my side, I believe I can find solace and renewal.

A note on birth

We often have a birth plan, either written down or in our minds, but you know what they say about best-laid plans! They rarely happen exactly as we intend, especially with birth because it's often a wild and untamed process. But plans create expectations, and when an outcome doesn't line up with those expectations, it can leave us with a feeling of grief or a sense of loss over how we *thought* the experience would unfold. Let me reassure you (in case you need it today) that the choices you made during your baby's birth were made based on information available at the time, and that is all you can do. My son's birth did include many of the elements I hoped for, but when I think back, I still shudder a bit with how challenging it was—how I was pushed to the very limits of my physical and emotional self. I still can't look at it straight on, as it's too raw; like the sun, it's too close to revel in continuously. Let this be a reminder that no matter how smooth or rough your birth experience, it may take time to alchemize the experience in your mind and body.

However birth unfolded for you, it was the chosen path of your baby—it's how they wanted to come into the world (however messy or confronting or complicated). You honored that by being their vessel and making the best choices you could in the moment.

When you were in your mother's womb, you got to choose how you wanted to come into this world. This time around, it was your baby's choice. So, let it be okay if it was different from what you expected.

(A PRAYER FOR TODAY)

God, give me comfort in knowing that whatever happened in birth, there are lessons to be learned and they are part of the story about how I got to meet my baby.

The ultimate transition

In an instant, everything changes, but at varying paces. A month ago, for example, you were a "pregnant woman"; today, you are a "mother." However, even with a swift title change, the recalibration required within your body, mind, and soul takes time. And that timeline looks different for everyone.

The journey to motherhood is an experience unlike any other—transformative, profound, and life-altering. It leaves a deep impact on a woman's psyche. When a woman becomes pregnant, there is a societal focus on the physical experience of motherhood because that's what the outside world can *see*. But the birth of a mother, as I am sure you can already attest, is about far more than the biological changes in the body. It is a transformation that touches every single part of your being. There was "before motherhood" and "after motherhood," a line drawn in the sand within the storybook of your life.

So, I want to remind you today to have patience with yourself as you stretch, shed old skin, and undergo this massive shift. So much of your identity is being redefined in ways you may not have expected, and it may take weeks, months, or years to step into this title fully. Know that you have ample time to find your footing as you embark on the ultimate transition.

(A PRAYER FOR TODAY)

God, thank you for entrusting me with the role of mother to my baby. May I remember that this new title reflects your boundless trust in me.

Sip of Self-Care:

Express gratitude to your body by honoring it. Set a timer for three minutes and stretch your body intuitively. Bonus points if you incorporate a foam roller into your stretch session. Throughout the day, ask yourself: "How can I treat myself more gently today?"

Heavy doesn't always mean stuck

Being the primary caregiver for another human being is an immense responsibility, and the weight of it can lead to what is often described as "nurture shock." This term captures the overwhelming nature of motherhood, where you may feel like you're teetering on the edge with balancing the endless demands of your little one, fulfilling a perpetual to-do list, and searching for time for self-care. It's a constant struggle between maintaining your composure and feeling like you're about to crumble. Yet amid the chaos, you uncover a wellspring of strength you didn't know you possessed. It's in those quiet, late-night cuddles, the small victories, and the pure delight in your baby's eyes that you find the courage to keep going. Even as you cling to the swinging rope of change, you discover that you're also learning to soar above where you have walked before becoming a mother.

Through each challenge, you cultivate a newfound grace and compassion, changing the way you see yourself. Keep moving forward, Mama.

Heaviness doesn't always mean being stuck; sometimes, it's simply a chance to embrace your own limits and grow.

(A PRAYER FOR TODAY)

God, on days where it feels hard, walk with me. Give me peace of mind, body, and soul. Help me find gratitude for the moments in between.

Calm environment = calm mama

Today, my mom came to visit and when she asked me how she could help, I blurted out impulsively, "Can you help me clean this place up?" I'm sure she was hoping I would have said something more like "Could you sit and stare at the baby while you rock him to sleep?" Either way, she obliged.

It took us twenty minutes. We put away the dishes, ran the vacuum, and threw the clothes that were tossed in every direction into one basket. Later, I decided to walk across the street to grab a small bunch of flowers. When I got home, I hummed in the kitchen as I bounced my baby on my chest and arranged the flowers in a vase. I lit a candle, burned a stick of palo santo, and sat down. As I looked around the room, I smiled. I breathed.

This exercise of tidying up the space (which was by no means perfect) was a mini reset. I immediately felt more at ease, and in turn, I could tell my baby did as well.

Where can you find a mini reset today? It could be as simple as playing your favorite song or lighting a candle.

(A PRAYER FOR TODAY)

God, I am so grateful for this home and the people in it. Give me a sense of peace and serenity as I go about my day.

The steady drum of your heartbeat

I first came across the fascinating concept of the imaginal discs of caterpillars in Lucy Jones's book, *Matrescence*[3], and it completely transformed how I think about continuity in growth and change. For a long time, scientists believed that a caterpillar, reduced to liquid goo in its cocoon stage, would emerge as an entirely different being—a butterfly—without any element of its former self. However, a 2008 study[4] revealed a much more fascinating reality: during this transformation, the caterpillar retains memories through specialized structures called imaginal discs. These tiny clusters of cells contain the blueprint for the butterfly's adult form and preserve neural connections, allowing the butterfly to carry memories and learned behaviors from its caterpillar stage into its new life. Even in the midst of total metamorphosis, something essential stays the same.

This continuity reminds me of how babies experience comfort and familiarity as they transition from the womb to the outside world. In the womb, your baby is soothed by the rhythmic environment created by your body—your heartbeat, your breath, the gentle motion of your movements. Some parents find that gentle, rhythmic patting on a baby's bum mimics this soothing rhythm, offering a sense of familiarity and comfort. Whether or not the science confirms this specific example, the truth remains: your baby carries with them a deep imprint of the environment you created within you.

Just like the caterpillar's imaginal discs, your baby holds a memory of you at their core—a memory of your steady love, your heartbeat, and the safe world you provided. It's a reminder that you, simply by existing, are a profound source of comfort and connection for your baby. Your fierce, strong, and loving heart has already made a lifelong impact on them, weaving continuity into their transformation from womb to world.

(A PRAYER FOR TODAY)

Thank you, God, for all the memories and for the gifts of health, well-being, and love. May I remember the love in each moment.

Who you are becoming is more than who you once were

Sometimes my mind flickers to the things I have lost since becoming a mother, sort of like the clips of a movie reel that remind me of a different time. Have I lost some of my freedom? Perhaps. The spontaneity and ability to stay up late bingeing a good Netflix show? Certainly. Have I lost some of my carefree nature now that part of my heart is swirling about the world outside of my body? Sure.

But I have gained so much more.

It's additive, regardless of how many times you are told (or how many times you feel) that you are losing some aspects of yourself or your life before having a baby. For if you add up what you are leaving behind compared with what you are gaining, you will always come out ahead because your wingspan is in expansion mode. This path of motherhood is a transformative experience that adds a whole new dimension of love and purpose to your life as it *widens the aperture* of your mind.

Through the turbulence of motherhood, we discover our inner strength, resilience, and a deeper understanding of ourselves. Ultimately, this can enrich and enhance every aspect of life, leaving a lasting imprint on our heart and soul.

(A PRAYER FOR TODAY)

God, thank you for who I have been. And thank you for who I am becoming. Show me the doors of expansiveness that are here and now, waiting for me to walk through them. All I need to do is be who I am now becoming.

Sip of Self-Care:

Acknowledge Your Presence

Each time you catch a glimpse of yourself in the mirror today, repeat the following words aloud:

"I love you; you are beautiful."

It may feel a bit funny at first, but as time goes on, it will be less awkward, and it's so wonderful for your child to hear you talking lovingly to yourself in this way.

Be where your feet are

Some days it can feel like we are stuck in a loop of changing diapers, feeding, and rocking. I've actually started thinking that God made it this way so we can excel in a few things early on and gain the confidence we need to find our footing as we enter motherhood. It's as if the menu was intentionally kept limited to eliminate the possibility of decision fatigue.

It occurred to me today that while the actions themselves may be similar, it's our state of mind that can give these activities a fresh flavor. Think of your state of mind as the toppings (sprinkles, chocolate sauce, nuts) to the vanilla sundae you are served each morning.

This concept has stuck with me throughout motherhood. In everything we do relating to our babies, it's not just about *what* we are doing but rather *the state of mind* from which we do it. So, instead of going through the motions today and using the time to think about the rest of the day or the next thing on the schedule, place your attention on the present moment and be (mentally) where your feet are (physically). See how this new bit of flavor tastes.

(A PRAYER FOR TODAY)

God, open my eyes to the magic in the mundane and grant me the willingness to experiment and play within my routine. Let me feel adventurous and spontaneous in my approach, knowing that the more I embrace the small moments in life, the more it opens to me.

It is both a blessing and a curse to feel everything so very deeply

In some ways, I feel more powerful than ever by bringing this baby into the world. In other ways, I feel deeply raw, vulnerable even, as if I opened a portal to give birth and it isn't quite shut yet. Simple things, like having more than a few people in my home, feel overwhelming. I often need to decompress once family or friends have left.

Do you feel this too?

Your heart is malleable, and your energy field is sensitive at this point. Be assured that this is normal and a beautiful part of the healing process. Taking your days as slowly as possible is key, and checking in with yourself when you feel prompted to leave the house or when you decide to let someone in will go a long way in protecting your peace. Saying no to anything that feels energetically draining is the biggest gift you can give yourself. Let go of the expectations to show up for anyone else except you and your baby in this sacred period. Also, build in time to decompress after interactions with people or any activities outside the house. Release any energetic debris they may have left behind. You are exerting so much mental and physical energy just by caring for yourself and your baby that the extras may just be too much. And that's okay, Mama.

(A PRAYER FOR TODAY)

God, give me peace today in knowing that I am doing exactly what I need to be doing. Let the rush of the outside world melt away from my mental sphere and send rest my way.

Amid the transitions, connect to what is unchanging

Autumn beckons us to let go. In the early autumn of motherhood, we are led into a continuous process of letting go of obligations, commitments, and priorities. We make space—space from certain relationships, from showing up in the way we once did, from answering emails and text messages with the same urgency as before. Just as leaves inevitably fall to the ground, we find ourselves in a steady state of nonattachment.

This "letting go" process is evident from the very start. What fits your baby loosely on the day of birth is too small in just a few short weeks. One day, out of nowhere, your little one smiles at you for the first time, says their first word, takes their first step.

It's not just newborn attire that teaches impermanence. All of motherhood is a lesson in it. You are continually letting go of your former self and surrendering to each new phase of your baby's development and your rebirth.

When the world around you feels like it's shape-shifting, the best way to anchor yourself is to connect to your innermost self, the *permanent part of you* that is unchanging. Whether it's a few minutes of closing your eyes and breathing deeply while you shower, or listening to your go-to morning podcast while you rock your baby to sleep, find the things that remind you of the parts of yourself that are in a steady state. This core does not shift with the seasons but remains constant through all transitions, guiding you through the beautiful impermanence of this journey.

(A PRAYER FOR TODAY)

God, connect me to my innermost self, the part of me that is unchanging amid the transitions of life.

Revel in being a magic mama

Your love is a transformative salve, soothing and renewing.

Your love is *the healing*. Nourisher, comforter, provider, protector, safe landing space, your baby's first earth, haven, playmate, best friend.

This is all you. The sacred frequency of mothering that pulses with empathy and compassion. For your baby, sure, but also for yourself. Revel in it. When you feel like your impact only lives within the four walls of your home, remember that it's so much bigger than that. Like magic, it's working in unseen ways. Your love shapes lives, mends hearts, and heals the world. It begins internally within you but love has eyes, hands, and legs and, sweet Mama, you are the embodiment of it.

This is the sacred essence of who you are. You are magic, Mama.

(A PRAYER FOR TODAY)

Let love be the medicine always, God. Teach me to walk in your love—in my thoughts, words, and actions. Always.

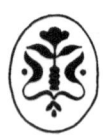

Sip of Self-Care:

360-Degree Breathing

Whenever you feel yourself overwhelmed today, lie on your back with one hand on your belly and one hand on your chest and take five deep breaths as slowly as you can. As you inhale, imagine the breath filling all around you—into your belly, ribs, and chest. Slowly exhale, releasing any tension. Continue this 360-degree breath, expanding in all directions, and feel the calmness flow through your body. Notice the difference even a few short rounds of breathing can have on your nervous system.

Friendships purified

Most big shifts in your life require a reckoning with the life you had before. In this period of spinning within the cocoon, it can be scary to let others in when you are still in the deepest parts of your transformation. When my best friend came to meet my baby for the first time, I felt both excitement and unease. I wondered how this moment would unfold. Would she see the ways I've changed? Would she understand how becoming a mother has reshaped me?

But as soon as she arrived, all of that faded. She hugged me, and I softened. She held my son with such tenderness, and I softened. She asked questions that felt genuine, listened deeply, and marveled at the little life I'd brought into the world. In those moments, I realized something profound: her love hadn't shifted—it had deepened. She wasn't just celebrating me as I was before, she was standing *beside me* in the person I'm becoming.

That night, as I went to sleep, I felt such gratitude. Gratitude for a friendship that could meet me in this new chapter with love and grace. Gratitude for the way she embraced my son as if he'd always been part of our story. Gratitude for knowing that some relationships, when tested by life's biggest changes, shine brighter than ever. Friendships, purified, is part of the process.

(A PRAYER FOR TODAY)

Help me feel at peace with the relationships in my life and bring forth those that are meant to be in this chapter with me. Let those relationships that are not aligned with this new version of me fall away with ease.

We break down to break through

Since becoming a mother, there is a part of me that feels that it's my job to be the "strong one," the one who knows the feeding times and routines. I am, after all, the one who birthed another human from her body. The role of the "protector" of my child came naturally and, with that, also brought more masculine elements of assertiveness, leadership, and sturdiness. But layered in the moments of feeling powerful were hues of anxiety and overwhelm. In between the moments of feeling so much love for my baby and this new role as mother, I have flashes, full-blown waves even, of feeling helpless.

On this night, I woke up at 3 a.m. and immediately felt the tears welling up in my eyes. I was confused by this because nothing specifically had happened to trigger the emotion. Rather, it was the weight of it all, the pressure of having it all together. It's as if pieces of paper were being placed on one side of a seesaw and eventually, that last piece of feather-like paper caused the whole side to plunge to the ground.

I felt embarrassed for a moment. What was I even crying about? But I let myself feel it. I went to the bathroom and let every tear drip from my eyes, for seemingly no reason. But when I was done and stood up, I felt clearer, lighter, and, honestly, very tired. I climbed back into bed and fell asleep almost right away. When I woke up a few hours later, I was grateful for that experience. It reminded me that often, what looks like a breakdown is really a *breakthrough*. We are crossing a barrier, which, although temporarily uncomfortable, is necessary for clearing out the old and making way for the new. In this season of Autumn, remember the beauty of letting go.

Growth requires release. Stability is not the absence of struggle, it's the ability to develop authority over the struggle. We sometimes must wade through the hard to get to the good.

(A PRAYER FOR TODAY)

God, let me release what wants to leave and welcome what wants to come. Help me live from full openness and trust that my experience is designed to lead me to a higher version of myself.

Welcome to matrescence

When I first saw the word "matrescence," I didn't know what it meant, but it resonated deeply. As I read about it in *Mama Rising* by Amy Taylor-Kabbaz[5], I felt an incredible sense of recognition, as though the word itself had been waiting for me. It stopped me in my tracks. Matrescence describes the developmental passage when a woman transitions through pre-conception, pregnancy, and birth into the postnatal period and beyond. It was the first time I had understood motherhood as a *journey*, not as an overnight sensation strictly tied with giving birth.

The term was first coined by Dana Raphael in the 1970s, but it has gained renewed attention in recent years thanks to Dr. Aurélie Athan[6], a clinical psychologist at Columbia University. Dr. Athan has been a powerful advocate for this concept, emphasizing the transformative truth behind her phrase "words create worlds." Without language to describe it, the experience of matrescence can feel isolating and vague, which is why reviving the term has been so impactful from a cultural perspective. It's also why I feel so deeply passionate about raising awareness about it now.When women recognize that what they're going through is not "just in their head," it can profoundly shift how they perceive their journey. It allows them to offer themselves more grace.

Consider this: Before the term "adolescence," people struggled to understand the intense and often disorienting changes in children transitioning to adulthood. Similarly, before "menopause" entered our vocabulary, there were countless unkind ways to describe the shifts women experienced as they aged. Shared language has the power to connect us, offering a framework to encompass deeply personal yet universal experiences.

Dr. Athan describes matrescence as a spiritual rite of passage from maiden to mother. And in case no one has welcomed you yet, allow me to be the first.

Welcome, Mama. So much growth and transformation awaits, and you are already on your way.

(A PRAYER FOR TODAY)

As I watch my little one grow and flourish, help me see my own growth and expansion as a mother. Give me the wisdom to trust my instincts and intuition, knowing that I can provide all that my child needs.

Rest: It's part of the process

When you're pregnant, your internal organs reorient to make room for the baby. As you know, it typically takes nine to ten months for this process; it's slow and intentional. After your baby is born, reorientation within your body occurs again, and similarly, that process takes time. Outwardly, you may appear "recovered," but within, layers of healing are still weaving themselves back together. Whether your birth was vaginal or cesarean, your body is a holy landscape in need of tenderness and time.

Consider this: It's no coincidence that our babies arrive unable to crawl, reminding us to pause and meet their stillness with our own. Rest alongside your baby. Take the day slower than you had planned. Rest is sacred. And rest is an act of faith—to surrender fully.

(A PRAYER FOR TODAY)

God, give me the wisdom to know my worth doesn't depend on how productive or task-oriented I am. You already created me inherently worthy. May I lean into the comfort of resting my body and soul.

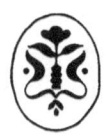

Sip of Self-Care:

Find Your "Rest" Language

Rest is as unique as your fingerprint. For some, it's a bath lit with candles and soft music; for others, it's thirty minutes sitting on the back porch taking in the outside air. Perhaps it's surrendering to sleep while your baby naps or saying yes to help when someone offers to tidy up or hold the baby. Whatever rest looks like for you, may it be free from guilt and full of grace. Listen to your body's whispers—they hold the blueprint for your renewal.

Celebrate how far you have already come

Over a whole month in, Mama. I'm sending you a warm smile and a hug through the cosmos. I want to celebrate you because if we wait for life to slow down before celebrating our journey, we might miss it. If we wait for the ocean to be still before we dip our toes, we may never have a swim. With each new birth comes a lot of change—in you, around you, and within your day-to-day.

Today, as you find yourself feeling around in the gray space of activity, I want you to take a moment and infuse joy into your day. This could be something as simple as dancing in your kitchen—or in the shower. Open the blinds, feel the sunshine on your face. Soak up the feeling of coziness that surrounds you. Call a friend (if you feel up for it). Lean into nourishment in ways that feel familiar.

(A PRAYER FOR TODAY)

God, let me see the light in myself, in my loved ones, in my sacred spaces. Thank you, thank you, thank you.

Uniquely yours

Sometimes it's easy to forget that our babies are their own person. They already have a personality with their unique sounds, coos, likes, and dislikes from the moment they are born. While we play a powerful part in shaping and nurturing these little lives, they shape us as well. I learned that my baby prefers sleeping on my chest and always runs warm, that when he feels a sacred line crossed, he makes it known through a loud screech (sort of like a pterodactyl), and that when he needs to go the bathroom, he has a blank stare on his cute little face. And it is my role to pick up on those cues.

Just as you are learning all about your baby, they, too, are learning about you—your smile, facial expressions, body language, and even preferred sleeping/feeding positions. And like all relationships, it takes time and observation as the new becomes *known*.

Similarly, you are getting to know yourself in this new role as a mother, as a woman in deeper initiation of who she is as a protector, nurturer, life giver, and soul stirrer. Be patient as you learn. Because in all of time and space, *your becoming* in motherhood is uniquely yours, like a fingerprint without a match.

(A PRAYER FOR TODAY)

God, may I always remember that though my children are born from me, they are not mine but theirs alone—their own being, their own person. Teach me to honor the divinity in them, just as they revere the divinity in me as their mother.

Your body hears everything your mind says, so tell a good story

As a mother, I also serve the roles of storyteller and narrator. I speak the words that describe what's going on in the world around my baby and me. One story I have been telling friends (and importantly, myself) is how much I have "fallen off" doing my daily practices in motherhood. Before my baby was born, my morning routine was full of juicy and nourishing emotional, physical, and spiritual well-being rituals. Now, there's just not enough time in the day with the demands of motherhood (or so I tell myself).

But today, after telling this story to my mother on the phone, I sat down to rock my son to sleep. As I did, I found my breath, closed my eyes, and focused on how much I love the feeling of his warmth and weight on my chest. I took a deeper breath, then settled into the chair and said a little prayer in the dark room. At that moment I realized I am still incorporating my practices into my life as a mother—they just look a little different now.

I may not squeeze in a Pilates class every day, but I am walking around the neighborhood while pushing a (very heavy) stroller. I may not be sitting down for a twenty-minute silent meditation, but I am taking mini pauses all day to reset my frame of mind.

We can get so stuck in how life is supposed to look that we create the narrative that we aren't doing enough, then allow those words to create our world. So today, let's worry less about what our routine looked like pre-baby and more about the ways that we can find small pockets of self-love rituals for our body and mind *in the season we are in.* Let's speak to ourselves with a sense of kindness as we build the storyline, one that supports our life as a mother.

(A PRAYER FOR TODAY)

God, allow me to appreciate the small pockets of peace and ease in my day. Remind me that my story is written by my words. Encourage me to speak to myself with grace and kindness as I build a new set of routines.

A note on co-regulation

When your baby is upset, staying calm can feel like an impossible task. Their helpless cries cause a cascade of reactionary hormones that send your brain and nervous system into overdrive, leaving you on high alert. Yet in these moments, your baby needs you more than ever; your calm nervous system is an anchor helping them co-regulate and find a sense of ease. It's a simple concept but one that can feel extremely challenging in difficult moments when you want everything and everyone to settle down, including yourself.

What is a small action you can take to regulate your nervous system? For me, its lightly tapping my wrist or gently tapping my baby's back with my two fingers when I'm holding him. Find something that brings you back to your body, grounding you. From here, your baby can use the soil of your nervous system to root theirs.

(A PRAYER FOR TODAY)

God, please grant me sensations of ease, calmness, and peace in challenging moments.

Sip of Self-Care:

Alternate Nostril Breathing

Set a three-minute timer and settle into a comfortable seat. Close your eyes or lower your gaze to soften your focus. Bring your right hand to your face and prepare for alternate nostril breathing, a gentle practice to calm the mind and shift your body from a fight-or-flight state into rest-and-digest. Put the three fingers in the middle of your hand down so just your pinky and thumb are sticking outwards.

1. Begin: Use your right thumb to softly close your right nostril. Inhale deeply and slowly through your left nostril, letting the breath flow with ease.

2. Switch: Close your left nostril with your right pinky or ring finger, release your thumb from the right nostril, and exhale fully through the right side.

3. Continue: Inhale through the right nostril, then switch again—closing the right nostril with your thumb and exhaling through the left.

Repeat this cycle at your own pace for the duration of the timer, focusing on the sensation of the breath moving through each side. Let your exhales be a little longer than your inhales, inviting your nervous system to unwind. When the timer rings, take a moment to breathe naturally, noticing how your body feels more grounded and at ease.

The fact that you are trying is enough proof that you are strong

The testament to your strength as a mother isn't your ability to get the laundry done while the baby rests. It isn't juggling all your old to-dos while keeping a tiny human alive. It doesn't depend on your lack of frustration while changing yet another diaper.

It is about something other than getting it right (whatever "right" means). Your strength exists in the moments of *trying*, in the consideration you take to ensure your baby is cared for. Your power is your presence, your observation, and your action when needed. It's finding the answers to your questions or calling the pediatrician at 3 a.m. because your baby made a strange noise and you just want to double-check that it's normal. Your power is in facing sleepless nights and days that simultaneously seem to drag on and flash by. It is a job we show up to even on days we don't feel like it. We do it anyway because we are strong.

Like the tall sturdy oak tree with firmly planted roots, you are unshakable, even in seasons when you feel like so much of yourself has fallen away, leaving you bare. There is something deeper within that is still alive and well, grounded and strong.

(A PRAYER FOR TODAY)

God, allow me to recognize my efforts are enough for my baby.

Closing the portal

Leading up to and during birth, a woman's mind, body, spirit, and auric field experience are all thought to be "broken wide open" to create the portal needed to usher a new soul into this world. We grow life in our womb and then bring forth that new life into the world. It takes extreme expansion to do.

But after forty-plus days, I felt ready to close this portal and put my walls back up, not in a bad or guarded way, but just enough to be a little more protected. I was ready to return to my center. My place of strength. So, my postpartum doula performed a traditional "closing of the bones ceremony" that included an herbal bath, a warming womb massage, and the tight wrapping of cloths over my body before saying a prayer. I was in a cocoon-like state. While wrapped, I reflected on what I wanted to trap/lock inside me from this chapter of birthing my son. And I spoke out loud what I wanted to leave behind, what I no longer wanted to hold. When the cloths were removed, I felt reborn in a new way, emboldened.

Whether you embark on a similar ceremony, I invite you to think about closing the portal and this chapter of pregnancy and birth as you step forward into your full power as "Mother." What has the chapter of bringing life into this world taught you so far? What feelings, experiences, beliefs, and ideas can you rid yourself of? What is ready to be given back to the earth?

(A PRAYER FOR TODAY)

God, thank you for the expansion and opening I have experienced in bringing my baby earthside. May I feel a sense of confidence and care as I close the portal. Pour your blessings of abundance and self-love over this closure, sealing it with love.

A field that has rested yields the most bountiful crops

No matter how much caffeine we consume, we still need rest. No matter how much we think we are used to operating these days on little sleep, we still need to reset. Rest is the body's way of refueling, and just like everything in nature, we are cyclical beings.

As a woman living and functioning in modern society, where everything is happening at light speed and you are required to be on the go all the time between social media, work, career, family, and friendships, partaking in rest is part of the *motherhood revolution.*

Gone are the days of over functioning, auditioning for the self-imposed title of "Super Mom" (picture the eight-armed mother sitting cross legged, trying to meditate, while her littles climb all over her while she juggles work, relationships, cooking, cleaning, parenting, and all that comes with the mother load).

You can end that pattern every time you choose to rest.

Some of the best initiations and creations in life require you to rest deeply, so rest when you are called to rest. Everything else will be there, but there is only one you. And you are of no good to anyone, including yourself, when you sacrifice rest and martyr yourself at the altar of people-pleasing, over-giving, and overextending your mental, emotional, and physical capacity.

Today, give yourself time to rest, no matter what that "rest" looks like. Stop. Breathe. You're enough just as you are.

(A PRAYER FOR TODAY)

God, give me the grace to accept rest as part of my self-responsibility. Just how nature has seasons, so do I. It is safe to rest. It is safe to allow my whole being to come to a standstill so I can hear your voice and be who you've called me to be.

Release your expectations to find something better than your imagination can create

I had many ideas about what I would be like as a mother long before becoming one. In my daydreams, I would move about the world with ease and grace, baby on my breast. Smelling the top of my baby's head, I'd feel nothing but gratitude twenty-four hours a day. I would get dressed every morning, and my hair would remain perfectly styled. I wouldn't bicker with my husband over trivial household tasks or whose turn it was to rock the baby back to sleep. I'd never be frustrated or annoyed with my experience. Maybe you also had some unrealistic expectations like mine, or maybe they are different.

It's been said that expectation is the root of all heartache. This is definitely true. While those dreams about who we wished to be as mothers are nice, the pressure and disappointment of not fully finding yourself in that reality can be painful.

You may not be the mother with washed hair (at this point, I wasn't), and you may not feel grateful when spit-up makes its inevitable way into your ponytail, but the reality is, your baby loves you for you, not the idolized version of you. You are someone's mother, someone's home, someone's universe. Your baby is thinking that they hit the jackpot of mothers right about now.

So, I leave you with this powerful truth to recognize: To become the mother you will be, you may have to let go of the one you imagined you would be.

Over time, you may even find your version of motherhood better than you imagined. Make room for this real-life version of you, as a mother, rising to this role in a way that God knew you would. Let yourself be surprised.

(A PRAYER FOR TODAY)

God, allow me to surrender myself to the version of me I am meant to be.

Sip of Self-Care:

An Embodiment Practice

Make a list of the top five feelings you want to embody as a mother. Think beyond goals or tasks—focus on emotions and states of being. Use descriptive words like "nurtured," "empowered," or "peaceful," that resonate deeply with how you wish to feel in your journey.

Once you've written your five words, place them on a sticky note somewhere you'll see them often—your bathroom mirror, beside your bed, or even on the fridge. Let this gentle reminder serve as a touchstone, guiding you back to your intentions amid the beautiful chaos of motherhood.

Answers come in stillness

There is beauty in the pause. There is power in stillness. I know our minds sometimes feel like a pile of leaves that has just been upended by the latest gust of wind. Our thoughts become untethered and float about, focusing on the piles of laundry needing folding, how the home needs more organization, or how there are a million tasks on the to-do list for the upcoming weekend.

And in those moments, I take the time to place my hand on my heart and take three deep breaths. I remind myself that there is so much beauty in this moment. I savor the ritualistic routine that has now become motherhood. I revere its sacredness. I know I can always come back to the present moment regardless of how long I've been taken out of it. That's all that matters. For me, and for you too.

You don't have to seek the answers, they will find you.

(A PRAYER FOR TODAY)

God, show me the magic in each moment, the gift in every pause, and the gratitude on days when it all feels absolutely mundane. This, too, is a part of a prayer I once prayed—to live the life I currently have.

You are a giver, so give to yourself too

What do you most need to hear today?

This was one of the questions I asked to the one hundred mothers around the world that I interviewed when writing this book. Sometimes we are waiting for someone else to say the words we need to hear, and while I agree that it can feel good to receive that outside validation, the truth is that once you identify what it is you need, you can give it to yourself.

So, what do you need to hear today? Here were the responses I heard most. And maybe you need to hear them too.

"You are enough."

"You are loved."

"You are whole, just as you are."

"You are incredible."

"Thank you for all that you do."

"You are leaning into your edges and learning every day."

"You are doing a really good job."

"You will get sleep again."

At the end of the interviews, I always liked to remind my fellow mamas that while it may feel nice to hear these words from someone else (a partner or friend), they are just as powerful when we say them to ourselves. Validating your own experience and celebrating your matrescence journey are important too.

Say these encouraging phrases to yourself whenever you need to hear them, Mama. That is the assignment today. Give yourself exactly what you need. You give so much, so give to your own heart as well.

(A PRAYER FOR TODAY)

Dear God, speak to me in every moment so that I may hear your voice and silence the negativity in my mind.

There is strength in your softness

It wasn't until becoming a mother that I found strength in my softness. It started with the new softness of my body that had carried a baby for nine months. I felt strange in this new physical form in the early days of postpartum. I also felt complete shock and awe at the pure power of my body bringing another human into this world.

It always made me laugh that my son would soothe himself to sleep by holding the parts of my soft belly that I once would have been self-conscious of. But I know now that soft can also be strong, like fluid waves that carve up rock with its consistency. I know now that the strength it takes to soothe a baby back to sleep quietly and patiently is unparalleled.

Your supple body is a haven for your baby to rest. Your warmth and physical touch are life-affirming for your baby. This kind of strength, the soft kind, runs counter to the popular narrative of the modern world, but the truth is, it's the most profound strength there is.

(A PRAYER FOR TODAY)

God, allow me to soften more to the experience of motherhood and find strength there.

Learn who you are; unlearn who they told you to be

One thing you will find no shortage of, during both your pregnancy and the time that follows, is people telling you how to be a mother. These well-meaning friends, family members, and even strangers will share their bedtime rituals, products they love, daily routines . . . you name it. They will tell you what parenting methods to use, offer medical advice, and give you books you didn't ask for.

The truth of motherhood is that it's a learning-on-the-job situation. No one can tell you what kind of mother you will be or what will work for your baby. It's a deep process of listening within and letting the voice of who you are be stronger than the voice of who others tell you to be.

(A PRAYER FOR TODAY)

God, may I recognize my true self and listen to my own innate wisdom.

Sip of Self-Care:

Close your eyes and place a hand over your heart. Breathe deeply and ask yourself: *What has motherhood revealed about who I am?* Write down the first thoughts that come to you—gifts you've uncovered, qualities you've reclaimed, or new ways you've grown. Then, write one thing you love about this version of yourself as a sacred reminder of how far you've come.

Savor your morning mug

Mmm ... smell that, Mama? That's the fragrance of your fresh morning mug of tea, matcha, or coffee asking you to take a moment to bask in its warmth. Savor the quiet around you, even if it's for a few blissful moments. Savor every sip. And as you take each sip, set an intention for your day. Envision how you want to *feel today*, what will bring you peace and joy, what will ground and anchor you.

Make your morning mug time a beautiful ritual that grounds you and your frequency for the day, that shields your energetic capacity and anchors you into a field of love, presence, and gratitude so that nothing and no one can shake you, no matter what comes your way.

Slowly sip that drink and awaken to the beautiful world that is your life.

(A PRAYER FOR TODAY)

It is always a blessing to savor the simple moments in life. Thank you, God, for the life I have, the breaths I take, the steps forward I make, and the human, woman, and mother you've called me to be.

Bubble of peace

In preparing for birth, I took a hypnotherapy course that spoke about how I could enter a "bubble of peace" once my labor started. The bubble of peace is simple: it's is an imaginary barrier that lets you invite in people, emotions, objects, ideas, or anything that feels supportive. If something doesn't make you feel good, safe, or loved, then it isn't welcome inside the bubble. For example, whenever fear arises, or an unwelcome thought, you kindly ask it to step outside of the bubble.

I have now taken this concept past birth into postpartum. For me, this means I've chosen to distance myself from certain friends and family members who don't light me up (or tend to pop my bubble). Sometimes, it's turning off the TV in the middle of a show that feels violent or shutting off the news that is making me spiral.

While this concept is a mental exercise, it's also based in the physical realm— you choose the environment you are in, the people and feelings you let into the space around yourself and your baby. It's okay to put up your boundaries. In fact, it's necessary. As new mothers, we are particularly raw, vulnerable, and openhearted. The bubble of peace is one protective layer while we are in this period. And it's a place that your baby will also revel within.

(A PRAYER FOR TODAY)

God, send my angels into my bubble of peace and help me sense, with a greater knowing, what things and people are meant for me in this season. Give me the strength to ask for what I need and create the boundaries necessary to protect me in this vulnerable state of transition into motherhood.

You are the nutrient-rich soil in which your baby grows

Wherever you find yourself today, let it be easy for you and for your baby. It can be as simple as taking fifteen minutes to get outdoors, either with baby in tow or for some solo time. Breathe in the fresh crisp air, as it will impact your energy and mood and nourish your spirit.

As you walk about the earth, take it in with your five senses. Allow yourself to inhale the light so you can be the light, and not just for your baby and your family, but for yourself. There is something magical about stepping away from the chaos and whirlwind of the day-to-day to feel the sunshine on your face, its warmth radiating through, as nature embraces you in her symphony. Cyclical, yet spontaneous. Energizing and calming.

A sacred remembrance that like nature needs the right alchemy to thrive and grow, so do you. It's from there that you and your baby can flourish.

(A PRAYER FOR TODAY)

God, help me remember to see the light within. To appreciate the light around me, and in others.

You didn't come this far to get this far

So often when we are in the middle of a journey, we forget to look up and look around, and then when we do, we may realize we still have so far to go. It can feel daunting. For this reason, I made sure that my husband instructed our birth team not to tell me how dilated I was in labor land—the numbers would mess with my motivation.

By now, you have changed countless numbers of diapers, and feeding your baby has become a full-time job. At this point, you may still need to figure out how to get yourself bathed, fed, and rested properly. But today, let me remind you that you didn't come this far to get this far. The road ahead seems long, but you are well on your way.

Practice makes progress, and you are progressing down this path of motherhood one step at a time.

Keep your head up, Mama. You're doing it.

(A PRAYER FOR TODAY)

God, please protect me as I make my way along the path of motherhood. Remind me to enjoy the journey through all the ups and downs.

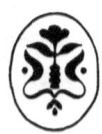

Sip of Self-Care:

Rooted Reflections

Journal to reflect on what has gotten easier over the last few weeks. Maybe it takes you half the time to change a diaper, or you've discovered the trick that lulls your baby back to bed. Congratulate yourself on three things, no matter how small.

The edges where I end and you begin blur and soften

In pregnancy, taking care of yourself, your body, and your mental health *is* clearly the way that you take care of your baby because of the obvious oneness between you. You eat healthy foods so your baby has nutrients; you walk outside and take prenatal vitamins that keep you strong to increase the baby's vitality. But don't be mistaken into thinking that this changes once your baby is earthside. There is still a oneness, an interconnectedness to the well-being of you both.

I realized today that I haven't washed my hair in over a week, my nails are broken from my relapse in nail biting, and I have been wearing the same leggings for two days. But my baby? He is glowing from his oil massage last night, he smells like oranges from the soap I bathed him in, he has a fresh diaper, he's been fed, and he's now grinning back at me with the cutest smile (albeit a smug one).

Even though you are now two separate beings, taking care of yourself *is* still caring for your baby because the way you feel, internally and externally, has a profound effect on the way you show up in your mothering. Additionally, it's important to show our children, from an early age, how it looks to love ourselves, to value ourselves. Gone are the days when we glorify the mother who has given all of herself to her children, and so much so that she doesn't have a drop left in her own cup.

You are an extension of your child. Your health and well-being will continue to be intertwined for decades to come.

(A PRAYER FOR TODAY)

God, remind me that I am also inherently worthy and valuable as a person. May I give myself the time and space to care for my own well-being, as I am an extension of my child, and our health is woven together.

Water what waters you

During pregnancy and early postpartum our brain is rewiring, and in this state of transient neuroplasticity, we are more susceptible to stress as our emotions and sensations are heightened. Everything we feel and experience is amplified. It's all normal, Mama. You are going through radical transformation in your Mother Year, the turbulent wind of matrescence at your back.

By now, there may be a familiar cadence to your daily routine, even if those routines are constantly changing, wilting into different forms as your baby goes through milestones or "leaps." There are so many sweet firsts that you don't want to miss; meanwhile, life tugs at you from both ends. You may be finding (as I have) that there is simply too much that is asking for your attention.

Some days, all of this can feel like leaves in a windstorm, tossed and torn in a tumultuous dance, struggling to find stillness amid the chaos. On these days, I invite you to sink deeper into moments of silence, taking deep breaths and grounding yourself. Letting each gust reveal the resilience and beauty within the tender, unwavering connection between you and your child. In the whirlwind of early motherhood, make sure to nourish yourself as you nourish your baby. It's not selfish, it's stewardship and self-leadership. You deserved to be watered too.

(A PRAYER FOR TODAY)

May my mind center on peace and tether to the parts of my journey that are sacred and nostalgic. Let my focus marinate on those parts.

Talk to yourself with love

Right now, we are feeling semi-settled in our routines, yet the nights are still long and the days feel choppy. I stay up all night and sleep sporadic hours during the day. Sometimes I look in the mirror and the first thought that flows through my mind is how tired I look, how dark the circles under my eyes are. And my reaction? Usually something negative like "Oh my, I look horrible!"

Yet when I reflect on it and catch myself, I remember that I never want my child to speak to themselves with a negative tone or to belittle themselves for anything.

It has been said that "it's not what is taught, it's what is caught." My baby is watching my every move; he is catching and learning what it means to be in this world from me. And that is a lot of responsibility and power that I am ready to hold and steward as a mother.

So today, I invite you to talk to yourself with love.

(A PRAYER FOR TODAY)

God, let my thoughts, actions, and words be a representation of your divine love and compassion. May I treat my mind, body, and soul with reverence. May I love myself wholly—in each season, in every moment—just as I want my child to love themselves.

The maternal circuit of your brain

These past few months have likely been a whirlwind of changes. You may feel different, and that's because *you are different* now, but the good news is that you are prepared for this on a neurobiological level.

Did you know that it's actually a myth that our brains deteriorate in motherhood? Studies have now shown that pregnancy and postpartum have a *positive effect* on long-term brain health. The hormones of pregnancy, birth, and even breastfeeding prime the brain to develop the "Mother Circuit," refining key areas of the brain in matrescence. Affected brain regions include those that enable a mother to multitask to meet a baby's needs, help her empathize with her infant's pain and emotions, and regulate how she responds to positive stimuli (such as a baby's coo) or perceived threats. Sure, we may feel foggy or forgetful at times, but that's because our brain is undergoing a process called "synaptic pruning" where the brain gets rid of weak connections to encourage the growth of new, stronger ones. Your brain is essentially rewiring itself to learn new, important skills. It's relocating resources to make itself brighter, stronger, and more efficient. How incredible is that? Your brain has been upgraded.

So, let's wear "mom brain" like a badge of honor moving forward.

(A PRAYER FOR TODAY)

God, thank you for changing me into the woman and mother I am today. Guide me to tap into all the ways I am prepared for this chapter and remind me that I am powerful as I raise the next generation of humanity.

Sip of Self-Care:

A Nod to Your Noggin

Each time you do something for your baby today, whisper the following words to yourself so that they become ingrained in your subconscious:

"My 'mom brain' is my superpower."

The sixth sense

We go about the nightly bedtime routine in joy—a warm bath and oil massage before nursing and settling into the chair I now know better than my own bed. We turn the lights low, and I sing in a soft voice, rocking back and forth. But as the evening stretches on, with my son's eyes *still* open ever so slightly, I find myself drifting to the list of things that require my attention.

And the more I want him to fall asleep, the longer it seems to take him to get there. I wonder if he knows. He must, I tell myself. It's as if he can feel the energetic pulse get louder and brighter as the to-do list items build in my mind. He can sense even my slightest shifts in mood. So, I stop *pretending* to relax and start doing it. I slow down my breath, I let my eyes drift closed, and I embody the calm that I am wishing upon him. And what do you know? He finally closes his eyes too.

I guess there are no secrets here, as he can spot all my tells.

What a gift, this sixth sense of his.

(A PRAYER FOR TODAY)

Thank you, God, for giving me this innate connection with my baby. May we attune to each other's souls and rhythms and remember that we are loved. That is what matters most. Everything else can always wait.

Motherhood as the equalizer

Before motherhood, I would have considered myself a generally kind and empathic person. But once I had a baby, those feelings were taken to a whole new level, and frankly, one I was not prepared for. Now I find myself seeing people, adults even, as a child of a mother somewhere, and I wonder what their journey was like. When I see unhoused people on the street, I wonder about their mothers and my heart physically aches for her and for them. When I see a mother at the grocery store with a crying child, I feel drawn to lend some relief. Where I once saw my role as one who cared primarily for herself, I now feel a shared responsibility to care for the collective. Maybe this is part of the village mentality. While it has become more diluted in today's society of "living in our own lane," it resides in us still.

I feel it rising within me more each day, because among all the things that motherhood brings, it also acts as the great equalizer. It gives us boundless empathy to see the good in others. We all began as babies, emerging from our mothers' womb. We were all born with soft skin and pure hearts.

Stand in awe of the web of the human experience that weaves through us all.

(A PRAYER FOR TODAY)

God, make me a channel and conduit of love, compassion, and kindness. Help me see you in every person I meet. My light is your light is our light.

Trusting love to lead

I see you trying to be, do, and carry everything.

Your partner attempts to help you, in their own way, and then you find yourself giving more direction, perhaps even redoing what they've already done. Maybe, just maybe, you hesitate to leave them alone with the baby because a quiet voice inside wonders: *What if my baby adapts to them and doesn't need me as much?* But the truth is, when we give our partners the opportunity to care for our baby, it empowers them and plants the seed of confidence that is vital for them to grow into the parent we want them to be.

Did you know the brain of a non-maternal parent changes too? But *only if they are regularly engaged in caregiving.* They must be involved for the physiological changes to take place. So, give their primal caregiving instincts a chance to flourish. Give your partner a chance to step up and embrace their leadership as a parent.

Will it be perfect? Probably not. Will it be exactly the way that you wrap your baby, or change their diapers, or soothe them, or bathe them? No. Maybe they'll put your baby in the wildest outfit you've ever seen (I've been there a few times). But it will be done with love and that love is what matters most.

Recognize the things your partner does well. The more you lift up your partner, the more they feel prepared (and inclined) to step in and be helpful.

Build them up so you can both rise together.

(A PRAYER FOR TODAY)

Thank you, God, for giving me a partner who is supportive, loving, and kind. Their way need not be my way but give me the patience to allow them to grow as a parent too.

Not a perfect person, but a perfect love

There have been so many times already on this journey when I have second-guessed myself, my decisions, my way of being a mother. I saw an analogy once that likened this position of motherhood to someone making you the CEO of a company that you had no prior expertise with—but hey, good luck!

In the past, I could research a topic endlessly and find answers, but in motherhood, there is so much that lives in the gray that has no "right" or "wrong" answer. It is less about solving the issue of the day and more about trial and error—what works for you and what works for your baby in this moment.

So today, as I found myself deep in another online forum, I heard a message from deep within whisper "Put down the phone." It was a reminder that what I was searching for wouldn't be found on the internet or in a book . . . it was within me. I may not have all the answers, but I love my baby in a way that no one else does or is even capable of.

I don't need the perfect answers because I have the perfect love.

(A PRAYER FOR TODAY)

God, remind me today that love casts out all fear and doubt over being imperfect. Remind me that perfection is not a way of being but rather the ability to love unconditionally. May I see the power within me and find comfort in the fact that you have appointed me as CEO of my baby.

Thank you for your trust.

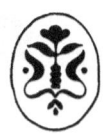

Sip of Self-Care:

Wrap your arms around yourself, give yourself a squeeze, and feel the immediate warmth and sensation of being held. Know that today, your presence is enough; the perfect love you have for your baby is all you need.

Let the trees remind us that growth requires release

This week I started to pump for a host of reasons, and I was surprised by how emotional it felt, and not because I was worried about my baby having bottles. I had this sense that I was losing something, namely my sole ownership over the feeding relationship that we had been doing for the past two months. My partner wanted to help feed our baby, as did my mother. In theory, these were welcome and kind gestures to give me more support, but something in me felt resistant to this change. Pumping allowed me to run errands without the pressure of needing to be back to feed a hungry baby, but as I ventured out, I couldn't help but feel a little lost. As I sat in my car, not really wanting to even go into the store, I realized there is a fine line between losing something and *letting it go.*

I was perceiving this extra level of help as a weakness, the partial loss of a role I held. As mothers, we often feel like we need to do it all, all the time. But letting go is required for growth. We will continue to shift and change routines many times over in our motherhood journey and unclenching our fingers around the situation and intentionally softening into the moment brings a lightness that otherwise is simply overshadowed in guilt.

Seasons can be long, and they can be short. And even within one season, therein lies many micro changes that happen that look like small losses or releases, depending on your perspective.

So today, I am taking a note from the trees around me and letting go of this feeling that is weighing me down and leaning into what newness this change surfaces in my life. I am moving forward with the gumption that I am doing my very best. And I hope you do too.

(A PRAYER FOR TODAY)

God, on days when it feels hard to release control, help me breathe and let go. I am worthy because you created me worthy. My worth isn't defined by what I do, how much I do, or how I lean into support. Give me the grace to appreciate every season, wholly.

Your well has no end

Thoughts from today that are on my heart:

In moments when doubt begins to rise within me,

In moments when my body aches in places I didn't know existed,

In moments when tears well up in my eyes,

In moments when an ache swells in my heart,

I remember, I remember—

The truth that as a mother,

My well of love, kindness, compassion, and patience runs deep,

So deep, in fact, it has no end.

Sometimes I just need to send the bucket back down to fetch a little more.

Our well never runs dry.

It's deeper than we know

We just have the send the bucket back down

Again,

And again,

And again.

(A PRAYER FOR TODAY)

God, in times when I feel my well is drying up, I turn to you for comfort and replenishment. Renew my spirit and fill my heart with your presence and love, reminding me that I am never alone or empty.

Marinate in the metamorphosis

In those moments when your baby is lying on your chest and the whole world feels quiet and calm, during those nights when it feels like everyone is sleeping but you are up rocking away, you may sense the metamorphosis that is upon you. You are expanding your wingspan, your mindset, and your heart space. You are shedding the layers that are no longer needed to make space for what is needed. It is in the stillness that we hear the whispers of our heart.

Between taking care of your baby, socializing, work, relationships, etc., the small voice within that you need to hear most can be smothered. So, rock a little longer, stare out the window, and listen to what she has to say. Your soul is always speaking to you. Sometimes in whispers. Other times in deep breaths. Soften to listen.

(A PRAYER FOR TODAY)

God, in moments when I forget to listen to your voice, to the voice of my soul, help me linger in the quiet moments a little longer. Help me attune to the whispers of my heart so I can make room for where I am meant to be. Help me soften into my becoming.

Let the spiritual undercurrent guide you

Life is inherently spiritual. Often, we get caught up in the minutia of daily existence and forget that it's all so miraculous. After all, we are made of stardust, particles born from ancient stars. In these early days of motherhood, it's easiest to forget this cosmic truth. This season is fleeting, yet it can feel all-consuming when you're immersed in the never-ending rhythms of baby care. But there is magic in the mundane, if you know how to look for it.

Did you know that a newborn baby's sense of smell is so finely tuned they can recognize their mother's scent from birth? This innate connection is part of the miracle of life itself. Can you shift your focus from the material to the spiritual undercurrent that belies it? The miracle of motherhood mirrors the miracle of life, each sacred moment full of wonder. When we are spiritually centered, we become less swayed by the emotional turbulence of the day. And it is this deeper undercurrent that can carry us further than we ever dreamed.

(A PRAYER FOR TODAY)

God, please reveal to me all the wonders of each moment.

Sip of Self-Care:

Held in the Sacred Moment

Place one hand on your heart and the other on your belly, feeling the rhythm of your breath and the gentle, steady beat of your heart. As you inhale, silently affirm: *I am woven into the fabric of something miraculous.* As you exhale, let go of any tension, overwhelm, or expectation, allowing yourself to simply be—fully present, fully enough, held by the sacredness of this moment.

It's called a season for a reason

Have you ever noticed how, during our highest moments in life, our minds automatically fear that the good times won't last or come around again, yet in the toughest moments, we convince ourselves that this will be our permanent reality? The truth is, both the highs and lows are temporary.

In motherhood, this fact can be comforting and daunting at the same time. We feel the weight of holding on to that sweet newborn smell or the size of those little toes, while also longing to sleep more than a few hours at a time. We are in a specific season of motherhood in this moment. So, whether you are still riding the newborn high or feel deep in the thick of it, just know that this is just a chapter in your life. It won't last forever.

Instead of wishing and waiting for the next phase, be here now. Just recently, an elderly lady walked up to me at the farmers' market. She smiled at me and simply said, "Babies don't keep."

A good reminder that yes, there is an expiration date to this version of us, my baby and me, and to this chapter we are living.

(A PRAYER FOR TODAY)

God, help me see the silver lining in all that is. I am grateful for the season I'm currently in, and I know this, too, shall pass and newer doors will open.

Bounce forward

Before I became a mother, I heard the term (and in all honestly, probably referenced it once or twice in my own plans) "bouncing back." As I sit here now, I realize what a misnomer it is.

Matrescence, as you may recall, is the profound shift that happens in your body, hormones, mind, and spirit when you have a baby. Some say it's the biggest shift we go through as human beings, akin to the process of adolescence—the transition from childhood to adulthood. Dr. Alexandra Sacks[7], a reproductive psychiatrist, underscores this parallel by highlighting that both stages encompass major hormonal-shifting and body-changing times.

Now, imagine telling a teenager that you can't wait to see them "bounce back" into being a child. You wouldn't. You couldn't. It's impossible. Once you have undergone such a monumental transformation, you are forever changed.

The same is true for mothers. We are never the same, nor should we try to be. Motherhood reshapes us at our core; we have new wisdom filling our bones. Even something as simple as how we dress can feel different AM (after motherhood). And that's okay. We're not "bouncing back." We are bouncing forward.

(A PRAYER FOR TODAY)

God, in times when I feel the pressure of returning to my former self, remind me that I was meant to undergo this monumental change and this new growth is all part of my path forward toward my purpose and in furtherance of a full and vibrant life that is meant for me.

Giving yourself space to grow

In the sacred journey of motherhood, the greatest gift you can offer your soul is the freedom to evolve and embrace the transformative waves that are settling deep within you. Create a nurturing space where you can unfurl your wings fully and step into your new roles: Mother. Protector. Guardian Angel. Problem solver, comforter, nourisher, and nurturer. Allow yourself to truly see who you are becoming.

Though your outward appearance may remain familiar, within you unfolds a profound metamorphosis. This evolution requires ample space to flourish.

Your love is a healing force. Embrace it, revel in it.

Did you know that the sound of a mother's voice can calm her baby's stress response? Research shows that hearing their mother's voice activates a baby's brain in ways that help regulate their emotions and reduce anxiety. This sacred connection is part of the profound transformation you're both experiencing during this time.

So, the next time you're feeling doubt, fear, or that negative voice creep in, be gentle with yourself. Hand on heart, whisper to your soul, "I know we're growing. We are reborn."

This isn't just your baby's time to grow and unfold into their newness, it's yours too.

(A PRAYER FOR TODAY)

God, let me see the growth in each moment, even when it seems mundane. Help me honor the woman I am becoming.

Parenting as a practice

As I was changing the thousandth diaper tonight, it dawned on me that there are parts of this experience that you can really get a hold of, like changing diapers or nursing your baby, but the journey of motherhood itself is and always will be a *practice*. And just like meditation or yoga, the goal is simply to show up time and time again, to allow the practice to reveal a new part of itself, and to encourage expansion and growth by taking you to your limit. By humbling you each time you think you have it "figured out."

For me, this idea of parenting as a practice takes the pressure off a bit. A reminder that showing up, day in and day out, with an open heart and curiosity is all that is required. I am meant to fall and get back up again. I am meant to try something new the next time having learned from the time before. I am meant to peel back new layers in this continuous learning mode. That's all, nothing more.

To commit to a personal practice in motherhood. That's my goal.

(A PRAYER FOR TODAY)

God, give me the humility to see motherhood as a practice, supporting and guiding me as I discover the different parts of this journey. Show me small signs today of your love and devotion to my ongoing evolution as a mother.

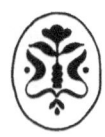

Sip of Self-Care:

Honor the Everyday Wins

Recognize and celebrate your accomplishments, no matter how minor they seem, in the practice of parenthood. Being a mom is a significant achievement in itself. Start a running list, either in a journal or on your phone to remind yourself of how far you've come and the strength you carry each day.

Here are some examples to get you started on your list of accomplishments in motherhood:

- Successfully navigating a sleepless night and still showing up for your little one the next day.

- Managing to get everyone dressed and out the door (even if it's a little later than planned).

- Giving yourself grace when things don't go perfectly.

- Asking for help when you need it and recognizing the strength in doing so.

- Creating a peaceful moment for yourself in the middle of a busy day.

Reset the alarm bells

We went on our first outing today where I was driving with my baby in tow. A friend of mine came along, and even though it was a relatively short drive around Chicago, within the first few minutes, my son started crying in the back seat. My friend seemed unbothered; she hummed sweetly, trying to distract him. But I could feel the heat rising in my body, the tears welling behind my eyes. His cry got louder and more pronounced (you know what I mean—when our babies really pick it up a notch). After a few minutes, I was so flustered, I pulled over, crying, and went to him. Had I not fed him enough? Was something hurting him? *Something* had to be wrong to warrant that cry, right? As soon as I sat next to him, though, he settled and even smiled at me. I checked the car seat, it all seemed right, and he was warm and fed. He just didn't want to be in the car, and he wanted his mother next to him. Completely understandable.

It took me some time to settle back down so we could finish the last five minutes of the trip, but I learned something: crying doesn't always mean that a baby is in need (which is what my nervous system was telling me). Now I'm not saying that we should let our babies cry, but I am suggesting a reframe for our nervous system in those moments when we can't get to them or when we feel overwhelmed, inadequate, or just plain old devastated because they are crying.

Babies only have one main communication tool and that is to cry. It doesn't necessarily mean they are sad; it just means they want something *to be different.* You are their problem solver and hear their "language" more acutely than anyone else. Next time you feel yourself flustered by your baby's cries, remember that it doesn't mean you aren't a good mom or that you aren't giving them everything they need. They just need something to be adjusted, and you are doing your best to figure out what that is. You are an amazing mother.

(A PRAYER FOR TODAY)

God, in moments of overwhelm, help me remember that this role of motherhood is a big job, but you selected me out of all the other people in this world because you know that I can do this. Let me find my breath and my calm so that I can respond to my baby's wants and needs.

This is both the destination and the journey

In my first thirty-three years of living, I was always striving, always looking to improve and be the "best" version of myself. So, when I became a mother, I thought the goal was to be the best mother I could be too. (Will someone be handing out gold stars?)

But the problem with becoming the "best" at anything is that it assumes there is a destination, something to eventually be achieved. That doesn't exist in our personal self-development, and it doesn't exist in motherhood. I have moments when I long for the day I will know everything I need to know. But the truth is, that day won't come.

Mothering is a lifelong course—there is always another class or credit to take to explore a new facet of the journey. Showing up to the "class of life" and squeezing out the learnings from each day is what motherhood asks of us in order to navigate the roads, rivers, and mountains that present themselves.

Where you stand today *is both the destination and the journey*. You are already here; you have already arrived. Let that sink in. You already have the gold star, Mama, just by being in it.

(A PRAYER FOR TODAY)

God, help me remember that where I am today and who I am today is enough. Let me see the goodness that you see within and give me peace to know that you are there every step of the way.

You will sleep again

At this point, I couldn't believe I had made it this long with such little sleep. I didn't know it was possible. But I find myself constantly learning new depths that seemed unfathomable a few months ago. Before becoming a mother, I needed a good eight to nine hours to feel rested. Now I would settle for a four-hour stretch. The truth is, though, that eventually whatever stage, leap, or change your babe is going through will end. This, too, just like everything else in motherhood, is ever evolving and therefore, temporary.

Did you know that when female flamingos have babies, their color turns from pink to white? The temporary loss of color is a testament to the flamingo's devotion and sacrifice. As their babies grow stronger, the flamingos gradually regain their brilliant pink. It is a beautiful reminder of resilience and renewal that reflects the cycle of giving and receiving.

You will sleep again, and you'll get your pink back too, Mama. I promise you that.

(A PRAYER FOR TODAY)

When I am feeling depleted, help me settle my body and mind so I can rest. Allow my baby to sleep and give me reprieve when I need it most.

You are the Mother of a lifetime

On the hard days

Easy days

Exhausting days

Fulfilling days

Beautiful days

Overwhelming days

And seemingly perfect days,

You were made to be their mom.

There is nobody more perfect than *you* to do this.

Your baby chose you. Their first choice.

For the woman you were and just as importantly,

for the mother you are becoming.

They hit the jackpot, Mama,

Because you are truly incredible.

You are the mother of their lifetime.

You both are on a lucky streak.

(A PRAYER FOR TODAY)

God, help me remember my assignment and initiation as a mother is a gift from you. You chose me to be the mother for my child. On days when it's easy to lose sight of this mission, help me remember that I was chosen for them.

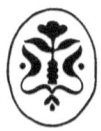

Sip of Self-Care:

Set aside ten minutes just for you—whether it's during nap time or with the help of a loved one caring for your baby. Use this time to reconnect with your body and energy. Start by jumping in the shower, letting the water wash away the heaviness of the day. If you have a gua sha or a dry brush, take a moment to gently glide it along your face or limbs, encouraging lymphatic drainage and releasing tension. After your shower, massage a nourishing lotion or oil onto your skin—arms, legs, and face—moving slowly and with intention. Slip into a fresh, comfortable outfit, then take a deep breath before returning to your baby. Notice how your renewed energy feels—it's not just self-care, it's stewardship of your body and mind; it's a ripple effect of light and love that radiates to them.

Beauty runs soul deep

Beauty is soul deep.

"Wow, she bounced back so quickly." We've all thought it, we've all felt it—the insane drive and desire to "bounce back" into our pre-baby body, our pre-baby energy, our pre-baby everything. The world seems to celebrate a quick return to the "before," as if that's the pinnacle of success. But what if the true beauty of this season lies not in the rush to reclaim the past but in the slow unfolding of the present?

I remember standing in my closet one morning, overwhelmed. My body felt new, foreign, still healing. Nothing fit—physically or emotionally. Tugging at clothes that no longer worked, I thought, *Who am I now?* I felt lost in a body I didn't recognize, unsure how to move forward.

I finally put on something simple and soft—something that felt like me in the moment, not me from before. I stood in front of the mirror and looked deeper. Past the body, past the awkwardness, past the stories I was telling myself. And what I saw surprised me. There was wisdom in my eyes that hadn't been there before, a gentleness in my heart that shaped the way I moved through the day. I realized I didn't need to rush through this transformation; my body was carrying me, just as it had carried my baby.

Postpartum recovery isn't a race, it's a metamorphosis that takes months, even years, to unfold. Yet we feel the pull to move through it quickly, missing the grace it holds. Today, pause. Look at yourself in the mirror and *really* see yourself. Your beauty isn't in the size of your jeans or how "together" you look. It's soul deep.

Give yourself time to revel in this transformation.

(A PRAYER FOR TODAY)

Whenever I feel like my body needs to do more, or be more, let me remember the power it already has within it to create, nourish, sustain, and grow life. May I always look beyond the surface and see the beauty in my soul and those around me.

Beware of "the compare"

Comparison can be helpful in some instances; for example, if we feel inspired by someone else's way of living and then use that inspiration to generate motivation to make changes in our own life. However, most of the time (especially in motherhood), comparison sucks the wind out from beneath our wings. I have found myself comparing my life now to my life before having a baby (spoiler: it looks much different). I am also just as guilty as the next mother of looking on social media and seeing how other mothers do one of a thousand things that I do differently with my baby. It usually doesn't feel good, that's for sure.

Last night as I sat rocking my baby, I imagined the day when my baby feels like they aren't as good as someone else, and it made my heart ache. What would I say to him if he was feeling "less than"?

I would want him to know that he doesn't have to be like anyone else, that he can find his own way, that he is perfect just the way he is, and that he should let his own heart be the compass of his life.

I smiled and thought, *I think it's time to give myself that same advice.*

(A PRAYER FOR TODAY)

God, allow me to feel into my wholeness. You created me worthy as I am. In moments when I get lost in the sea of comparison, let me remember that who I am is enough.

Nature's playground

There are a plethora of clichés relating to motherhood, but not many things on this journey are universal because our babies are all different, as is our alchemy of circumstances and personalities. However, there is one secret relating to our babies whenever they are having a hard moment that works almost every time: Step outside.

Your baby is part of nature, and they come with an innate recognition of their counterpart—the natural world. I have yet to meet a baby that is not enamored with the sky, the trees, the wind, all of it.

At this age, your baby can see most clearly the colors green and red, two colors that show up often when we are in nature. So, step outside and find comfort in nature's playground today.

(A PRAYER FOR TODAY)

God, thank you for the gift of nature, with its beauty, wonder, and abundance. Let me introduce my child to your creation, Mother Earth, with ease, finding solace, inspiration, and gratitude in its every form.

Nurture a kind inner voice

During this time, everything is new. You have a new baby, a soul in your charge, in the most delicate physical form. At the same time, you are a new mother in a new physical form of your own. Here is my invitation: Can you be as tender with yourself as you are with your baby? Can you nurture your kind inner voice the way you would with your baby?

In moments of unsureness, it can be easy to ask whether you are doing this right. You may even wonder if you are enough. *Why haven't I figured this out yet?* you may question. These thoughts can be overwhelming. Instead, see if you might cultivate a beginner's mind. You are new at this, after all. It's only been seventy-six days. How can you soften yourself to the awe of the experience by cultivating curiosity instead of judging yourself for all that you might have left to learn?

(A PRAYER FOR TODAY)

God, grant me the grace to be gentle with myself as I experience the newness of being a mother.

Sip of Self-Care:

Tongue Scraping: An Ancient Practice

Begin your day with the ancient ritual of tongue scraping, a simple yet powerful practice rooted in Ayurveda. Using a tongue scraper, gently sweep from the back of your tongue to the tip, clearing away the buildup of toxins and stagnation accumulated overnight. As you rinse the scraper, envision not just your mouth but your mind being cleansed—making space for clarity and kindness to flow.

This act of clearing your mouth is a symbolic reset, nurturing a compassionate inner voice. As you continue this practice, let it remind you to speak to yourself with the same care and love you would offer to your child: gently, tenderly, and without judgment. Start fresh, not just in your body, but in the way you meet yourself each day.

Motherhood is not a one-size-fits-all

I have a few items of clothing that are labeled one-size-fits-all. It can be nice at times to have a T-shirt or jacket that isn't tailored to any one body, but imagine if your entire wardrobe was that way? How frustrating would it be to wear clothes that are made for the average human, with no part of them feeling like they were made for you? It sounds uncomfortable and unflattering, to say the least. Instead, don't we love those pieces that fit us perfectly, hug us in the right places, and bring out our best qualities?

Remember, motherhood is not a one-size-fits-all approach. It's completely natural to find yourself comparing your experience to others, but every mother's path is unique. Your baby is unlike any other, and the challenges you face are your own. It's meant to be that way. So, when you read things on social media or consume books on sleep, feeding, diapering, nursing, even soothing, you are likely to get a wide range of ideas and beliefs because there isn't one approach that works across the board.

Embrace your unique journey and know that you're giving your baby something truly special: your love and care. Don't be too hard on yourself. We're all learning as we go, and that's okay. Reach out for support when you need it, and remember, there is no right or wrong way to be a wonderful mom. That's up to you to define.

(A PRAYER FOR TODAY)

God, teach me grace and acceptance, especially in moments when I doubt the path I am on. Let me remember that my child chose me as their mother for a reason. And that for them, I am the perfect mother. We are learning and growing together. And when it feels hard, let me know that I am supported in each moment.

The inevitable ego death

For me, a big part of my ego was tied to the "people pleaser" within. I prided myself on being the person that people turned to for advice, the "really good friend," dependable, the one who remembered every important date and went out of their way to make sure everyone felt loved and cared for. These roles fed my sense of self. Once I had my son, though, something shifted.

I no longer had the energy to keep it up. More than that, I lost the desire to even show up in that way. Even the act of holding emotional space for others felt like too much at times. That part of me had faded, and in its place grew something deeper, something I didn't need to prove. I was filled with the fierceness of caring for my baby, of wanting to be present within my family unit. I no longer felt the need to give pieces of myself away easily or quickly, driven only by the pull of wanting to please. My tiny human needed me, and that was enough.

Another layer of my ego was the illusion that I had control over my life. Early on, I realized that my best-laid plans often unraveled before my eyes. I had to lean into the discomfort of uncertainty, a place I had tried to avoid before becoming a mother.

In this season of Autumn, we witness the wilting of parts of our lives; but remember that rebirth always follows. The burning away of one aspect leaves space for new growth in its wake—an invitation for what's alive within us to one day flourish bigger than what was possible before the burn.

So today, notice how you have shifted and changed. And know that you were meant to.

(A PRAYER FOR TODAY)

I release the parts of me that once felt beloved but now no longer nurture the woman (and mother) I am becoming. It is safe to be who I am at this unfolding in my life.

A word about our bodies

As I've mentioned before, I have witnessed so much rhetoric around "bouncing back after birth." Lately, I have seen a wave of culture countering that idea, one that can make you feel guilty for even thinking about the appearance of your body. You may have seen messages encouraging women to simply be grateful for the miracle their bodies are capable of, in bringing life into this world. For me, neither extreme fully resonates. I don't feel the need to return to any specific body image, but I do want to move forward with my health—balance my hormones, regain energy, and rediscover the sheer joy of movement.

Our bodies are beautiful because of the stories they hold. And your body, Mama, has the storyline of growing, birthing, and loving your baby. So be kind to yourself; it's okay to want to feel what you feel, whether it is a desire to move again or a need to rest in this period of softness.

Whatever you're experiencing, honor it.

(A PRAYER FOR TODAY)

Dear Body, I love you. I am thankful for you. Thank you, God, for being the truth in my body—in how she moves, loves, sustains, nurtures, and is there for me and my child unconditionally. Much like your love.

Anything can be a chance to connect if you let it

Anything can be a chance to connect if you want it to be, if you let it. This idea completely shifted my idea on caregiving activities like changing diapers, feeding, and clothing my baby. We can rush through these things, seeing them as tedious tasks, or we can see them as a chance to connect. Caregiving activities, especially in these early months, are where most of our time is spent, and for our babies, represent the most important things they are doing in a day. Reframing my approach in this way has made our days much more interactive and, in fact, has created less down time with space to fill.

For example, for diaper changes, see how it feels to:

- Warm your hands by rubbing them together.
- Make eye contact and signal to your baby what is about to happen.
- Take a deep breath (especially if your baby is crying).
- Speak each step out loud in a calm voice before picking up or moving your baby.

Try to move one beat slower than you want. Our default speed as efficient adults is much quicker than our baby's desired speed.

(A PRAYER FOR TODAY)

God, show me the gift of connecting in each moment. The surroundings don't matter because there is always room for more compassion, kindness, and gentleness—with myself and others.

Sip of Self-Care:

Reflect and Honor Your Growth

Reflect on the ways your life has changed since your final month of pregnancy. How has your body transformed? Your hopes? Your priorities? Write down five differences you notice and honor the growth within you. Today, let this reflection remind you that direction matters more than speed. Slow down, let go of urgency, and savor the connection in these everyday acts. You're building something beautiful, one moment at a time.

The weight of it all

I recently read a post about how it's not a break from our child that we crave but rather a break from *making decisions* that affect the whole household. This idea felt so alive for me. It's not my old life that I miss, it's the framework of my decisions being simpler with little-to-no impact on anyone else but me.

These days, the reality is that it's just not as easy to head out for a quick nail or hair appointment at the last minute. There is a web of decisions and planning that would go into this. Childcare needs to be sorted and directions given. Sometimes it feels like more work than it's worth to navigate everything for some time for self-care or a simple indulgence.

But as much as your decision to take time for yourself affects the household, your decision *not* to carve out the time has an even more detrimental effect on the long-term health of the family unit.

It's not an either/or. You can choose caring for yourself *and* caring for your child. When you are feeling like it's all too much, communicate with your partner or family member. Lessen the load. Many hands make light work.

You don't have to carry it all alone.

(A PRAYER FOR TODAY)

May I have clarity on how best to care for myself while also showing up as the mother I want to be. Give me peace and ease on this windy path.

Rest is the best self-care there is

Rest is a four-letter word for mothers everywhere. When anyone offered me the sage advice to "sleep when the baby sleeps," I thought about how I could possibly sleep when the laundry was piling up, meals needed to be made, and messages were waiting to be answered. And don't forget, I also have a career and passions vying for my attention. Plus, the reality is, some babies just don't sleep that much. I felt my eyes rolling before they could even finish the phrase. But honestly, there is some truth to it, and here it is: You should rest when you can. Rest doesn't have to look like a long nap or a perfect night of sleep (though wouldn't that be nice?). One of my favorite voices in motherhood, Zoe Blaskey, author of *Motherkind*[8], redefines self-care as energy management rather than an elaborate checklist. And rest is a form of self-care. Maybe that means zoning out to your favorite show while you rock your baby to sleep. Maybe it's asking someone to hold the baby so you can take a long, hot shower. Or maybe it's simply allowing yourself to put down the to-do list, close your eyes for a few breaths, and feel the weight of the moment lift.

The to-do list will always be there, and motherhood doesn't come with clock-out hours. But amid the endless tasks, there is beauty in choosing to simply *be*. Rest doesn't mean you're failing—it means you're honoring the season you're in. Find the quiet moments and let them hold you.

(A PRAYER FOR TODAY)

God, let me find pockets of rest in small moments to sustain and nourish me.

Flexibility is your new best friend

By now, you have already seen your fair share of changes, and it's only been a few months. I am sure you have noticed practices or ways of interacting with your baby that worked last month no longer do the trick now. It's because your baby is changing so rapidly. So, what does this mean for you, Mama?

It highlights that your greatest skill will be your ability to adapt, to not cling to any one chapter too tightly, to allow your mothering to be flexible. Choosing flexibility over rigidity will make you resilient in the face of everyday change. And things really do change overnight in baby land so approaching it with curiosity will make the transitions easier for your whole family. After all, it requires far more energy to cling tightly than it does to witness the waves and allow them to carry you.

In motherhood, flexibility really is your new best friend.

(A PRAYER FOR TODAY)

God, help me flow through the daily currents that might take me by surprise. Let me remember that to continually grow, we must change over and over again, and this is by your perfect design.

Your new seed of self

When you become a mother, it's like the tree of your former self drops a seed that represents a new version your life. And from that seed grows a lush, green sprout. It's a version of the tree, *but it's not the same.* Therefore, when you try to return to the woman you were before, the routine you were accustomed to, or the exact body you had before motherhood, it's like trying to put that new foliage back into the seed. It can't be done because the new life has already sprouted and begun to take root. Thus, I invite you to stop trying to replicate what you had before. Instead, let's nurture and protect this new seed, tend to her changing priorities and shape-shifting body. There is a beautiful life ready to flourish as the mother if only we can see it.

(A PRAYER FOR TODAY)

May I continue to embrace the growth that is being asked of me—from my soul, my body, and my mind. May I embrace each season for the beauty that it is.

Sip of Self-Care:

Water Your New Seed of Self

Grab a small towel and run it under hot water, then wring it out. Lie somewhere comfortable and drape the cloth over your face, on your chest, or over your belly—wherever feels good. For a little extra love, dabble a few drops of lavender or eucalyptus oil on the towel. Allow the warm towel to encourage your body and mind to soften and surrender.

Mirror, Mirror, what do you see?

Within seventy-two hours of being born, babies start using their mirror neurons. Mirror neurons are cells that hardwire us to mimic expressions and behavior we observe in the people around us. They are the initial road map for learning emotions, and it's how we develop empathy and sympathy for others. Babies are looking to figure out the world based on cues given by their caregivers.

So, we get to show them:

what love looks like . . .

what joy sounds like . . .

what safety feels like . . .

. . . just by moving slowly around them, making eye contact, smiling, or chatting with them in a normal, calm voice.

How amazing is that?

(A PRAYER FOR TODAY)

May I be a channel of love, of joy, of peace, and of childlike wonder. May I be the mirror that reflects my child's inner divinity back to them in every thought, every word, every action.

Inner peace is the new success

One of the most significant shifts I've experienced so far is the reordering of my priorities. Before birth (while I was patiently awaiting my due date), I had lots of time, energy, and the will to call friends, check social media, and respond promptly to texts. Basically, I was adept at handling just about anything that came my way. But now, everything has changed. My world is centered around feedings, nap times, and the needs of my baby. What once felt imperative, what once felt crucial, now fades in the background. Right now, nothing seems more important than the well-being of this little one in front of me.

So, what does a "successful" day look like now? Inner peace is my new benchmark.

Can I breathe through hard moments and savor the sweet moments when my baby is sleeping in my arms? Can I quiet my mind enough to notice the small details, like the scent of my baby's head or the gentle hum of his breathing as he sleeps? When I'm doing those things, I'm in alignment with my highest mother self, and there's no better feeling. There's nothing the outside world can provide that I can't find right here within my heart, a heart that beats louder and brighter with more love for this baby and this life with each passing day.

(A PRAYER FOR TODAY)

God, allow me to feel a deep sense of calm and peace washing over me. Open my eyes to the wonders of motherhood's daily ins and outs and help me feel awe and gratitude for what my life has become.

Deeply connected

I am proud of myself today for the simple fact that I have created a deep connection with my baby. And so have you. Look how much you have learned. You have absorbed so much this season, from the practical parts of being a mother (changing, feeding, nighttime sleeping, napping) to the spiritual and emotional side of motherhood. You stand in stark contrast from the woman you were just three months ago.

In case no one has told you today, you are doing a good job, and you are doing important work—work to shape the next generation of human beings. By infusing your little one with love, you are leaving your imprint on this world in more ways than one.

Deeply connected babies make secure, confident adults, and you are setting the tone every morning you wake up and care for your little one like you do.

(A PRAYER FOR TODAY)

Thank you for this gift of motherhood and the leadership that stems from it. Thank you, God, for making me the creator of legacies, forger of changemakers, and conduit of your love here on earth.

Learn to lean on

Before my son was born, I took a lot of pride in my independence. Although married to a wonderful man, I still interacted with the world as a sovereign being and felt like I could do most things "on my own." That all changed for me in motherhood.

Even with a partner who did 75 percent of everything that was unrelated to breastfeeding, I was initially disheartened by how hard it was to keep up with the unending, humbling, and overwhelming responsibility of caring for a baby. Here I was, this "strong" woman who could be brought to heaving sobs after ten minutes of my son screaming in the back seat of the car. This idea of pushing through and just "leaning in" didn't do it for me. I needed to "lean on" instead—lean on my partner, our parents, our friends, and the kindness and labor of strangers-turned-angels. I learned to put aside my pride and let people in. I have never looked back.

There are things that only you can do and then there are tasks others can accomplish for you. Notice the difference and delegate where you can. You don't have to do this alone—you weren't meant to.

(A PRAYER FOR TODAY)

God, thank you for the people in my life who love me and want to be there for me in my time of need. Help me remember that these people are my angels. Allow my heart and mind to open to let them.

Sip of Self-Care:

Connect with Your Village

Motherhood is a journey best shared, and building connections with those who understand your path can be transformative. Spend five minutes today exploring local in-person or online support groups or Mommy and Me classes to share experiences, seek guidance, and build connections that can help support you during this transformative period. Some of my dear friends came into my life this way.

Take this small step to find your village—you never know what beautiful connections might blossom.

What you focus on grows

For me, it's the little things that make me feel undeniably joyful. I keep think-ing how much I love my son's little smile when he is half-asleep, how he looks at himself in the mirror with such wonder, how good I feel after I meditate. It's what I focus on, what I choose to focus on, that grows exponentially. This doesn't mean that there aren't sad days or days when everything feels like I am rolling a boulder up a hill. There are many challenging moments in this season. Yet in these little moments, I come back to my breath, to my child's smile, to his every action that is so full of playfulness—it's a childlike sense of wonder and awe.

This practice reminds me of the withering burn of a bonfire. As we fix our gaze on that fragile glowing ember, its warmth requires our devotion of breathing life into it. With each breath, the ember pulses, drawing in the air, and in that attentive stillness, it begins to swell and dance. Eventually, flames leap and twist, transforming the ember into a roaring blaze, a testament to the power of focused intention and the quiet magic that turns a single spark into a radiant display of light and warmth.

Because what we focus on grows, and what we give our energy to gets bigger and brighter. You have that power, Mama, to keep warm when the cold starts creeping in. Notice what you are placing your attention on today.

(A PRAYER FOR TODAY)

God, help me focus on all that is good in each moment and appreciate all that is still a work in progress. I am a masterpiece in the making. It is safe to be who I am.

Everything we do for our babies comes from love

I know it's incredibly hard to hear your baby cry. As mothers, we instinctively want to soothe them, wishing we could wave a magic wand to bring them peace and happiness all the time. When our babies cry, our bodies respond by releasing cortisol, the stress hormone. This natural surge of cortisol underscores the deep biological bond we share with our babies. It heightens our protective instincts and sharpens our awareness, preparing us to meet their needs.

Through this journey, its important to what's yours to carry and what belongs to your baby. You can establish the perfect bedtime routine or create an ideal sleep environment, but ultimately, it's up to your baby to sleep. You can offer milk from your breast or a bottle, but it's up to your baby to drink. You can provide options, but it's your baby's choice and we must honor that without taking it personally.

We can only do so much before we need to let go of control and find peace in knowing we are doing everything we can. If your baby is safe, take a moment for yourself to reset and reground if you need it before returning to work together. They're developing their unique personality each day, and you are both evolving together.

To your baby, you are everything. You are love. Remember that everything you do for your baby comes from love, especially in those moments when it means just caring for them with an open heart.

(A PRAYER FOR TODAY)

I am love. Love is the highest frequency. May my child feel this overflow of love in all that I do and all that I am as we grow together.

(Winter)

BECOMING THE MOTHER

THE SECOND QUARTER:

DEATH, REFOCUS, RECALIBRATION

*"And that's what winter is,
a reminder that not all growth is visible on the surface."*

*Scan for meditations to guide you
through this season*

Winter: Becoming the Mother

DEATH . REFOCUS . RECALIBRATION

In this season, you begin to emerge out of the newborn forest.

The initial rush and shock of being a mother has subsided enough for you to dip your toes back into your world that existed before your baby was born. For some, this may mean returning to a profession. For others, it may mean getting out of the house more often or reconnecting with friends you haven't caught up with in a while. After months of the daily cycle of feeding, changing, and caring for your little one, you may feel restless. Or you may be navigating something big with your child, or you may be finally finding your stride with your baby. Whatever Autumn entailed, know that it brought its lessons and now, we move to Winter.

Winter is centered on rediscovering yourself, which calls for introspection and solitude. It's an opportunity to shine the metaphorical light—your attention and awareness (which have been primarily focused on caring for your baby)—on your own life as well. You are, in essence, widening the aperture.

In Winter, many women experience a sense of divide. During the first three months of our Mother Year, there's often a grace period when partners, family, and friends give us space to be "in the zone." But as we move into the Winter season, the expectations to reenter society, return to old roles, and reconnect with the life we once knew can feel overwhelming. We are no longer the same person we were before motherhood, so how can we simply slip our feet back into the old shoes? They no longer fit.

I vividly recall having a group of friends stay for the weekend with us during my Winter season. I felt nervous and unsure of myself. I knew they loved me and my baby dearly, but I also knew so much had changed the past few months. I questioned whether they expected me to be the same person. As the weekend unfolded, I was reminded that it was okay to show up as my new self. I journaled about how I'd felt held, how my friends had provided a loving, nurturing, respectful environment. And seeing them embrace my baby—ah, the tears are flowing as I write this memory. This is what we need in this season: the ability to show up as our renewed selves and feel accepted, loved, and supported for who we are *now*.

But I want to be honest, this won't always be the case. Not every encounter will be as welcoming. Often, when we return to work or social settings, people hold on to the person we once were. They don't allow space for our evolution, and that can be difficult to navigate. In these moments, we are faced with choices. Perhaps a job no longer serves us; perhaps some friendships feel disconnected. Winter calls for the deepest inner work in our Mother Year because we are reconciling who we are now with who we were. How do we want to show up? Where do we want to spend our time? What dreams remain important to us? What is collecting in our heart space? Many women make hard choices during this season, including separating from friendships or leaving jobs that no longer feel in alignment.

So, in this season of recalibration and rediscovery, I invite you to bring in the outside world only when it feels nourishing and warm. In your Winter season, you plot and plan, perhaps even try things on, but then step back inside, to re-center when needed. This is a period for deep recovery and preparation for the Spring that will come.

Pushing on the walls of life in the Winter season of our Mother Year may feel a lot like being a bird ready to hatch. There are moments when it feels like the world you knew is crumbling, and that can feel scary. But once you break out from the old shell, you begin to see the light and you stand up, breathe in fresh air, and marvel at how you ever managed to fit in the egg-shell at all. Allow yourself to be reborn into a life that serves your renewed self. For while your former versions of self are loved, and are a part of your evolution, your new form is the most powerful and most aligned version yet. Build your life around what serves this version of her instead.

In this Winter season, I offer these words to hold and guide you:

- We are always evolving, and with new chapters comes new adventures.
- What is right for you will show itself.
- You have the power to make hard choices.
- Only you know what feels right for your life.
- It's okay to feel conflicted.
- Take the lesson, leave the details.
- There is nothing more courageous than healing.
- You have time, so allow this process to unfold in its own divine alignment.

You've got this, Mama.

There is a magic to winter

In nature, it's easy to associate winter with death. The leafless trees lay barren, and there are no visible signs of growth. But there is a magic to winter. The quiet calm of potential is buzzing beneath the ice and decay. The death of what was is making room for what's to come.

One of the most difficult aspects for any new mother is the process of grieving their old life. It is simply a part of the initiation process of becoming a mother that we must then mourn the maiden. There were surely beautiful aspects to the life you lived before becoming a mother. It's okay to mourn the time you had to care for yourself or get copious hours of sleep, but remember to surrender to the season before you now. You may spend your current days in a bathrobe with your baby nestled like a starfish on a rock, always seeking your warmth and sustenance. Or you may be struggling to recalibrate as you return to work or step back into your business. Remember that is only a season and if it doesn't feel sustainable, that's okay because it's not meant to be. The sprouts of what is to come are hidden beneath the information you are taking in now. The magic is there, even if not yet seen.

(A PRAYER FOR TODAY)

God, allow me the space and time to properly grieve the life I had before I became a mother so that I may find celebration in the mother I am today and the life I am co-creating with my baby.

Peace begins with you

Where does peace come from? Have you ever wondered? It's certainly not made in a warehouse or manufactured in a shop. No material item can give it to you. Peace lives *within* you, and while certain people, places, and thoughts can help bring it out of you, you always have unfettered access to it at any time. How powerful is that?

As you breathe in deeply, close your eyes. Let the swirling thoughts of uncertainty and overwhelm settle. Breathe out and let it go. Repeat the words "peace begins with me" as you place your hand over your chest, holding your own heart. Feel empowered as the *"peace maker"* in your life.

(A PRAYER FOR TODAY)

May I remember that peace begins with me. It is always within me, no matter the chaos that swirls around. In each moment, I am PEACE. I am empowered. I am grateful. Thank you, God.

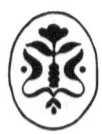

Sip of Self-Care:

Sacred Clearing with Sage

When life feels turbulent and your energy is scattered, turn to sage—a sacred tool used for centuries in many cultures for cleansing and renewal. Sage, especially white sage, is an herb traditionally burned in a practice called smudging, believed to clear negative energy, purify the air, and restore balance to both your environment and your spirit. You can find sage bundles at natural food stores, metaphysical shops, or online from ethically sourced suppliers.

To begin, light the tip of a sage bundle and let it smolder, producing a gentle smoke. Move the smoke around your body or space with an intention to clear away heaviness and invite in calm. As you do, repeat this affirmation:

"I am vaster than the waves of this moment. I release what no longer serves me and call in peace, clarity, and calm."

Let the practice center you in the present, reminding you of the deep, unshakable peace within you. When you're ready, safely extinguish the sage by pressing it into a fireproof dish, then carry your renewed energy forward.

Surrendering is powerful, and love is one form of surrender

The love we embody as mothers is unlike any other. It's palpable because it springs from a deep raw surrender. In this love, we embrace selflessness while remaining firmly rooted in the essence of who we are as a woman and mother.

This transformation happens when we release the need for things to be different from what they are. We let go of our thoughts of the future and allow ourselves to be fully rooted in the present moment, knowing that while we cannot control every outcome, we can control who we are in each moment, how we show up, and how we respond. It becomes a conscious choice—one that includes course-correcting when we feel misaligned.

Allowing all emotions to surface frees us from stagnation and opens us up so we can lead from our heart instead of our head. It also leads to less struggle, a clearer path forward, and the motivation to take action toward what we truly desire.

In essence, this period of surrender is simply love, unfolding in its fullest, most radiant form.

(A PRAYER FOR TODAY)

The Serenity Prayer attributed to theologian Reinhold Niebuhr reminds me to come back to grace, acceptance, and surrender during moments when everything feels like an uphill climb.

"God, grant me the serenity to accept the things I cannot change, courage to change the things I can, and the wisdom to know the difference."

A note on the decisions around work

This week of my Mother Year, I was scheduled to return to work—and it was soul-crushing. My whole life, society told me I should strive to be "successful," and I was by typical standards. I pushed myself relentlessly to excel in college, then law school. I poured years of my life into firm work with grueling hours before finally pivoting to philanthropy law—a path that felt meaningful. It was a career I truly loved.

And then I had a baby. After my son was born, everything shifted. I couldn't imagine sitting at a desk again, away from him. What once felt fulfilling suddenly felt impossibly heavy. Maybe you've been here too. That persistent voice in your head asking: What will happen to my baby when I go back to work?

Whether you're returning to work or are able (or have chosen)to stay home longer, give yourself grace. Wherever you are on that journey, you will find your rhythm, just as you found your way in those early, blurry days of motherhood. It may not happen overnight, but it will come.

And when the weight feels too much to bear, lean on your community, ask for what you need, and advocate for the space to figure it out. These decisions—how, when, and whether to return to work—are deeply personal, and only you can make them.

For me, I did go back to work but it took time to find a balance that felt right for our family. Some days it's still hard, and I remind myself constantly that it's good for my son to see me pursuing something I care deeply about. These choices carry immense weight, but with time and reflection, they'll become part of a story that feels uniquely yours. One day, you'll look back and see how beautifully it all unfolded.

Trust that you are on the right path, even when it feels uncertain.

(A PRAYER FOR TODAY)

I trust that everything is unfolding in perfect timing. I am always exactly where I need to be.

In the darkest winters, new life is still growing

I remember one particularly cold night (the kind where the cold seems to seep into your bones), the weight of everything felt unbearable. My son, just a few months old, stirred in his bassinet beside me. Exhausted and raw, I picked him up, his tiny body radiating a warmth that somehow reached the frozen corners of my heart. He rested against me, and in that quiet moment, I felt it: a glimmer of light breaking through the shadows.

Those days often felt like a dark night of the soul—an identity crisis so profound I wasn't sure I'd ever find my way through. Motherhood had cracked me open, and I didn't know who I was anymore. But as I cradled him that night, I realized something extraordinary. Even in the depths of transformation, life was blooming. He was blooming. I was blooming. Ever so slowly, we were expanding to find our way together.

When it feels like the darkness will never lift, search for the glimmers.

Cradle the new life budding in the cocoon of this Winter season of your Mother Year. In those fragile moments, you're not just surviving. You're acclimating. Recalibrating with intention. Evolving, together with your baby, with your family, and with your soul's purpose.

(A PRAYER FOR TODAY)

Show me the glimmers during each day and night. Thank you, God, for every single soul who brings light into my life.

The magic can't leave you when it's within you

There is still a lot of recalibration in your mind and body during this period. New neurons are creating new connection pathways. Your brain is shifting, and changes are upon you. You are cultivating a new depth of emotions, possibly a new network of friends, and a deeper connection with yourself, your body, and your baby. You may even have a new type of connection with your partner and/or loved ones (also, it's totally normal if that is not the case).

Many new mothers envision the first year of their baby's life to play out in a certain way, but that rarely happens. What we *can* control, however, is holding space for the evolution of our relationships. We need to allow the ones that will naturally grow *with us* to deepen and release the ones that are meant to naturally run their course and fall away. There are also some relationships (like your marriage) that may have felt effortless before but now need more intentional devotion and communication in order to thrive. Remember, the most important connection you will ever have in this life is the one you have with yourself and God. Those connections serve as the soil in which all other relationships are planted.

On days when you feel "forgotten," know you're not. You matter because it all starts with you. To those two little eyes that follow your every move, you are their world. To the soul within you, you are the magic. And the magic can't leave you when it's within you.

(A PRAYER FOR TODAY)

Thank you, God, for the village of support and love surrounding my baby and me.

Sip of Self-Care:

Even though you're now a mother, it's important to have moments of alone time to continually connect to the evolving version of yourself, as it can help you maintain a sense of individuality and recharge your energy. Ask your circle of support today for at least ten minutes to be alone or take time during baby's nap for some reflection time about how far you have come, what you're feeling, and where you're being led.

More will be revealed in the unfolding

Your deepest growth takes place in moments of vulnerability, moments when you are wondering if you left your phone inside the fridge yet again (true story!), moments when you question whether your baby is really crying (or whether you are imagining it), or in moments when you are finally away for an hour by yourself and you miss your baby so much. These are moments of growth; you're dancing the fine line of being a mother and being a woman in the midst of an unfolding transformation.

Motherhood isn't always about outward growth—it's more like gold, buried beneath layers of dirt and dust, waiting to be uncovered. With every challenge, every tender moment, the layers of who you are begin to shine through. The beauty of motherhood is not always instant—it's found in the sifting, the learning, and the gradual unveiling of your own strength and wisdom, one piece at a time. The more we lean into the mess, the more we discover the brilliance underneath.

Embrace the lessons that surface in each of these moments, whether it's a lesson on being present, breathing more, releasing control, holding boundaries, or giving yourself grace. There's a blessing hidden in each vulnerable moment waiting to be discovered. Lean into it. Get curious to see what you can learn from it.

(A PRAYER FOR TODAY)

Thank you for the grace in every moment. Thank you for the lesson in each moment I feel doubtful or fearful. Thank you, God, for walking with me.

A note on friendships

Who do you want to connect to today? Who's on your mind? Lean into the support systems that have sustained you through challenges. Take a moment to send them a text. Let them know you're thinking of them.

On this journey of motherhood, we meet new friends and deepen old friendships. We can also easily slip into a cocoon where we feel like everyone else should be checking up on us. In these moments, remember that we are all human. Give yourself and your support system grace. Check in on *each other*.

Lead with kindness—for yourself and others. Lean on each other. Steep in gratitude and send some loving energy their way while enjoying a hot cup of tea or relaxing in the shower. Wherever you find yourself, know that you're not alone on this journey.

(A PRAYER FOR TODAY)

Thank you, God, for surrounding me with old friends and new friends and all my loved ones. I am grateful for every single one of them.

Be still to reveal

Some days can be physically exhausting, always anticipating the needs of your baby. On other days, you may find yourself moving more in flow at a slower pace. Still, your thoughts may be constantly in motion. Much of the journey of early motherhood can feel like you are inside a snow globe, with a whirlwind of emotions, activities, and ideas swirling in your mind. But the beauty in the snow globe is not just the swirling snow, it's the picture underneath that we wait in anticipation to see. So how do we see it?

We stop moving the globe long enough to allow the sediment to fully settle. And when we do, we finally catch a glimpse of all that is happening around and within us. We can then see and appreciate the strong, beautiful mother who is growing every day.

(A PRAYER FOR TODAY)

God, thank you for getting me through each day. Help me see each moment not only for what it is but also for what it can be. Let my spirit be still so I can see through it all.

Create your soulful sanctuary

Don't be afraid to create new rituals that bring you joy. It's easy to get stuck in the day-to-day. Eat, sleep, clean up, diapers, meal prep, shower (if you're lucky), repeat. I know, I've been there.

On days when it feels like everything is a blur, I commit to a micro dose of my favorite rituals such as participating in prayer or meditation, doing a few minutes of breathwork, or going outdoors for a walk. And sometimes I'll add a new ritual that fills up my soul, be it reading from an inspiring book, listening to a podcast episode, or venturing to a new place in town with baby in tow (either just us or with a fellow mama friend).

There are no rules for these rituals. They can be as short as they need to be, just small bursts of self-care to break up the day. Create your soulful sanctuary whenever and wherever you need.

(A PRAYER FOR TODAY)

Teach me to lean into the new, to explore the road less taken. God, give me the grace to walk in faith and to trust in the newness unfolding for me.

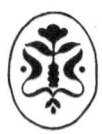

Sip of Self-Care:

Create a Heart-Centered Ritual

Transform a moment of self-connection into a sacred ritual. Find a quiet space, if possible, and light a candle or diffuse a soothing essential oil to create a calm and nurturing atmosphere. Place your hands gently over your heart, close your eyes, and take three deep, intentional breaths, grounding yourself in the present.

As you breathe, repeat these affirmations aloud (or silently), letting their truth resonate within you:

- "I am enough exactly as I am today."
- "I am growing, learning, and becoming every day."
- "I hold space for both my strength and my softness."
- "I am worthy of love and kindness, starting with myself."

To deepen this ritual, choose a meaningful object—a crystal, a journal, or even a favorite trinket or piece of jewelry—and hold it in your hands as you speak your affirmations. Imagine it absorbing the energy of your words, becoming a talisman of self-love and empowerment. Keep this object nearby to remind you of your inner strength whenever you need a moment of reconnection.

Rituals like this are powerful reminders that you are always worthy of care, compassion, and the time it takes to honor yourself.

As seasons change, so do you

You're in a new season of motherhood, already past the three-month mark. In this Winter season of your Mother Year, however, the nights may continue to feel long. I had many revelations and reflections that surfaced in these late, quiet nights when the world was still but I was up, rocking my sweet little one under the stars. In particular, my mind often wandered to memories that had long been buried—ones from my own childhood. I spent many moments thinking about my mother and other female elders in my life who've come before me. There was a newfound grace and patience in witnessing my own evolution that allowed me to more clearly witness the evolution of these women. Had they felt this way? Stretched and pulled? I suddenly had more compassion and could see how their story may have led to mine. There was something deeply humbling in witnessing my own evolution alongside the echoes of theirs.

In moments of doubt, remember: As the seasons change, so do you. Give yourself grace to witness your evolution. I am honest with friends and family about how my plans are likely tentative. I don't know how my day will look or how I might feel. I am in a season where I need flexibility and grace from the people around me. And so are you.

You are allowed to shift, to grow, to change course as needed. Your evolution is beautiful, even in its messiness. Trust the process—you're becoming exactly who you're meant to be.

(A PRAYER FOR TODAY)

God, grant me the courage to embrace my evolution. Give me the grace to witness the season I'm in and the knowledge to understand that this, too, shall pass.

Realize how little is needed, and you will always have a lot

It's okay to crave simpler moments.

By now you may be knee-deep in working, juggling multiple roles, and finding your groove. And you are missing the time at home with your little one in your arms.

Or perhaps you are shouldering all the mothering at home, a role that can be both challenging and heartwarming, and you miss the days when the weight didn't fall squarely on your shoulders at every turn.

You may even miss the simplicity of the moments before motherhood—the moments of pregnancy bliss before your baby arrived earthside, the moments when you had more time to yourself or control over your schedule.

It's okay to crave these moments, Mama. And it's okay to find joy in the simpler moments of motherhood. Notice what you are craving, then think about how your ideal scenario for work and mothering would look. And start to name it, out loud.

Today, give yourself the grace of keeping it simple where you can. There is power and elegance in that.

(A PRAYER FOR TODAY)

Reveal the beauty in the simple moments to me. Send a sense of contentment to my heart wherever I am, in each task that I am doing, in each conversation. Allow my mind to settle and hold on to a sense of peace. Remove any debris from my life that is not for me.

You are the hope

Do you remember the first time you held your baby? That moment when their tiny fingers wrapped around yours like a quiet promise? In that instant, you became their whole world—the answer to every prayer they couldn't yet speak.

I pray you always see yourself that way.

You are the light, Mama. You are what your baby prayed for. You are the mother your family needs, the partner your partner leans on, the friend who lifts others up, the daughter who carries the strength of generations before you.

I pray you see that you are the hope, not because you have all the answers, but because you show up with love, day after day. Just as you see the beauty and inner divinity in others, especially your baby, may you always recognize that same sacred light shining within yourself. You were made for this.

(A PRAYER FOR TODAY)

May I see, feel, and know hope every single day when I look into my own eyes, into my beautiful baby's eyes, and into the eyes of every single soul around me. We are here. Hearts beating, hope radiating outward. Every day is a miracle that I get to live out.

Find your "why"

What are your intentions as you settle into motherhood? Of course you want to be a good mother, but what makes a "good mother" in your eyes? I encourage you to start as you mean to go on. The early days of motherhood are a time to lay a foundation, and this intention will be your anchor.

I think back to a morning when my baby was only a few months old. I had just made it through a sleepless night, the kind where you feel like your body is running on empty, but you keep going anyway. I sat down to nurse him, and my mind began to race with all the things I should be doing (answering emails, washing dishes, folding laundry). But then, as I watched him gaze up at me, I realized this moment was so much more than checking items off my to-do list. He *needed* me, and my job wasn't just about getting things done, it was about being present with him.

In that moment, I made a quiet decision to prioritize presence over perfection. It became my "why"—to be fully there, in each moment with him, even when everything else felt chaotic. Sure, there would be days of exhaustion and self-doubt, but reminding myself of this intention gave me the strength to stay grounded in my purpose as a mother. No one can tell you exactly what your child needs, because no one knows them like you do.

Define your intentions, and let them guide you as you make decisions, big and small. When life feels overwhelming, your "why" will always be the compass to guide you back to what matters most.

(A PRAYER FOR TODAY)

God, help me discern what is for me and what is not. What is for my baby and what is not. Teach me to lean into your guidance as I continue to trust my own intuition.

Sip of Self-Care:

Creating a Family Intentions Space

Transform this exercise into a tangible ritual. Gather meaningful items—a photograph, a special stone, a small plant, or a written affirmation—that symbolize your values and vision. Arrange these items on a small surface in your home to create a dedicated family space.

Spend a few minutes each day or week at your space, reflecting on your intentions and reconnecting with your purpose. As you do, silently or aloud, reaffirm your commitment to nurturing a family rooted in faith, love, balance, and clarity. This special space will become a living embodiment of your heart's vision, reminding you of the beauty and purpose in your journey.

Let the sunlight wash away the old stories

At this point, the nights may still feel longer than the days. For us, a stretch of sleep is still quite a treat, and I take one whenever I can get it. But no matter how long the night was or how many times I was woken up by the needs of my baby, there is something about the sun rising in the morning that comforts me. The gentle light, when all is still and quiet, serves as a reset, like a blanket of freshly fallen snow covering the struggles of the night before. Whether I've been at my limit physically or mentally, when morning comes, it's a chance to begin again. Each day I remind myself that I am growing wiser; each day I further embody the *Mother*—surrendering, unlearning, relearning, and ultimately, transforming a little at a time. These elements are shaping us into a new form entirely.

(A PRAYER FOR TODAY)

God, let the morning sun be a reminder each day of your love that cloaks me and my baby. Let it remind me that you are always here, unwavering, to give me strength on this path of motherhood.

Anchor back often

What do you anchor into daily?

I began working with a lactation consultant when I noticed a troubling pang of emotional heaviness each time I nursed. It would fade, but I wondered if it was "normal." I soon learned I was experiencing dysphoric milk ejection reflex (DMER), a condition affecting some breastfeeding mothers that brings on a sudden wave of anxiety or sadness during the milk letdown phase. Though it only lasts for the first one to three minutes of feeding, for me, it often became a painful reminder of my internal struggles. While there's no cure, my lactation consultant encouraged me to discover something I could tether to, and not just in these hard moments while breastfeeding but also during the waves of motherhood that would continue to rock me at various points in my journey.

Some days, I anchor into deep breaths, finding comfort in the steady rhythm of inhaling and exhaling. On other days, it's the soft glow of a favorite candle, the soothing scent of an essential oil, or having my favorite tea nearby (peppermint) that provides a grounding sense of calm. These are more than an indulgence, though; they are tools that ease my heart and nervous system, offering brief but treasured moments of respite.

Finding our anchor helps us focus on the glimmers of hope and the small magic in each day. Whether through deep breaths, movement, calming scents, or quiet moments, these practices allow us to shine and show up with hope, even on the most challenging days.

(A PRAYER FOR TODAY)

God, you are my anchor. I see you in every person, including myself and my baby. In my loved ones. In the grocery store clerk. In the children on the playground. In other parents around me. In nature. In all the blessings I have. Thank you for surrounding me in every direction.

Which is harder: floating or sinking?

Isn't it interesting that when we are swimming and trying really hard to remain on top of the water, constantly moving our legs and arms, we will inevitably become tired, but as soon as we lie on our backs with eyes to the sky and lungs full of air, we float? The more we focus on not sinking, the harder it becomes, but when we utilize the resources within us (such as our breath), it becomes easier and more effortless to stay afloat.

In the same way, as new mothers, it's easy to believe the effort we expend directly correlates to the outcome, but is that really the case? I have found that doing more doesn't always produce better experiences, for me or my baby. What if you let things flow just a little more today? What if nap time starts a bit later than planned? What if you don't get to shower but spend a few minutes putting on a face mask as you go about your morning? What if you let the day take you in the direction it wants to instead of swimming against the current? You may actually feel better. Try it out today.

Allowing your day to be flexible, and soft, without expectations, is the easiest way to feel like you're floating rather than sinking.

(A PRAYER FOR TODAY)

God, help me go with the flow and find peace in the twists and turns that present themselves.

Your legacy starts now

If you could share anything with your baby about this time, what would it be? How would you describe this very moment to them a few years from now? Some people believe that babies are too young to remember details, but I believe these moments are actually the roots of their childhood, their life.

It may not always be obvious, but we know from nature that not everything has to be seen for it to be working. Think of the quiet of winter. Beneath the frosted earth, roots continue weaving their tiny tendrils deeper into the soil. While not visible above ground, these growing roots whisper a promise of spring, knitting strength and resilience in preparation for the seasons ahead. In the same way, these seemingly small moments, these memories you are making with your child, serve as their foundation. They are the delicate roots of their life, tethering to your loving relationship.

The days might feel long right now, but they will pass. And in the seasons to come, you will look back with gratitude on the strength and bond that this time has nurtured.

(A PRAYER FOR TODAY)

May I embody my role as both the creator and the coauthor of my life story with you, God. Together, we write our story, our legacy—as a mother, as a woman, and as a family.

Sip of Self-Care:

Set up an email account for your baby so you and your family can send notes to that inbox throughout their life. Set a reminder on your phone to send a short email every few months and encourage your friends and family to do so as well. You can even attach funny or memorable photos. When they open it one day, they will have a treasure trove of words and stories that will live on.

Find your people and hold them close

If you have ever felt like the village has disappeared, it hasn't. It just looks different now. In pregnancy, I had imagined attending Mommy and Me yoga classes each week with my baby strapped to my chest and having lunch dates with friends where we shared stories about the current milestones of our babies. However, I had my son in the height of the COVID pandemic. Thus, most places were closed, and social gatherings were essentially nonexistent.

So, I connected with a doula who was launching a virtual six-week post-partum mothers' class. I was nervous, but I signed up. I rolled out my yoga mat in my living room and adjusted my camera so I could breastfeed my son in private, if needed. As we introduced ourselves and started to share, something shifted in me. The words that flowed from the other mothers on the call spoke deeply to my soul. I was not alone.

At the end of the course we shared our contact information, and I keep in touch with many mothers from that community to this day.

The village is very much alive—it just may come in forms you weren't expecting. You may have to reach out, sign up, or subscribe. It now lives in community events or on digital platforms. It also resides within your local businesses and brands that have missions to support mothers.

Who is a part of your community, your inner circle? Your doula, your best friends, your family, your neighbors? Our village exists all around us if we open our hearts to new connections and, perhaps, unlikely relationships.

Babies, businesses, and families are not meant to be raised alone. It takes a village to not only raise a child but to raise *up a mother*. Find yours and hold them close.

(A PRAYER FOR TODAY)

Thank you, God, for my village. For all the ways they show up to support me. May I, too, be a source of strength and support for them.

Hibernate and say hello to the new you

I find that I sometimes don't have the energy, the will, or the desire to do the things I once did. I feel so guilty about that. Before giving birth, I journaled about the fear I had of losing myself. So, for a while, I held on tightly to the person I was before motherhood. I tried assuring everyone, including myself, that I could still be the same person. But I was different. My priorities were different. And I wasn't losing myself, I was gaining a new version of *me*. I was discovering inner terrain I had never traveled over before. When I finally understood this principle and gave myself the grace to shed my old skin, I felt a massive weight lift off my shoulders.

Expectations—we all have them for ourselves and others. However, how much freer would you feel if you simply gave yourself . . . permission to evolve. Permission to set down what no longer feels in alignment. Permission to choose new priorities—yourself, your baby, your family, your health, and your well-being. Permission to be who you are being called to be in this new era of your life.

Doesn't that feel amazing? Good. Consider this permission to hibernate and get to know the new you, Mama.

(A PRAYER FOR TODAY)

Help me release the things that are no longer meant for me in this season of my life. I bless and release it all with gratitude.

You are a walking, breathing, living miracle

Can you believe it? Your body has the ability and God-given power to grow, sustain, birth, and nourish new life. That is nothing short of miraculous. It's magical. It's sacred.

On days when you find yourself looking in the mirror and focusing on that pimple that may have popped up, or obsessing about the postpartum hair loss that continues, or on any ways your body may have changed, take a moment to pause and remind yourself of this: You are a walking, breathing, living miracle, Mama.

You were reborn with the birth of your baby. Your identity is shaped from the inside out. Forever evolving. You are the miracle that compounds and the life source that nourishes and keeps on giving.

(A PRAYER FOR TODAY)

Thank you, God, for my breath, my health, and my creativity. And most of all, for this sacred initiation of motherhood. Thank you for the daily doses of divinity I see in each moment.

Groove to the music

Find ways to move and groove in your day.

What's your go-to song to dance to? I've started cultivating some playlists that match the vibe I want to create, depending on my mood and the energy I want to infuse into each moment. To make it even easier, I've labeled my playlists by mood (ex: "upbeat" or "in my feels")—both for quick access and to give my husband helpful insight about how I'm feeling!

Studies show that families who dance together experience less anxiousness in their children. Why? Because dance helps release stagnant energy from the body. Sometimes there is nothing as cathartic as a kitchen dance party with your baby in your arms. When life is life-ing, do a little dance. Let the music move you. Find ways to move the energy through your day. It doesn't need to be a thirty-minute workout—it can be as simple as a dance to your favorite song!

(A PRAYER FOR TODAY)

Teach me how to dance when the ground feels shaky. Teach me how to dance and gracefully navigate each moment with calm and joy.

Sip of Self-Care:

Put your baby in a carrier and set a timer for ten minutes. Listen to a few of your favorite songs and let your head, hips, arms, and legs move freely. You can also listen to the music through headphones so you can really crank up the volume and get lost in the beat if that feels supportive (I've done this a few times during my baby's naps).

Your body, the temple

Your body is a temple. Think how you housed a tiny human inside your womb. Your body was their source of nourishment, sustenance, and comfort, and not just during pregnancy, but after.

Your body is not only your baby's first home and sacred temple, it is also yours too. Speak to it with gentleness, with love, with kindness. Gaze at it with pride, love, and grace every day. Feel your scars—they're golden rays of hope, proof of life lived.

Your body is your God-given temple. Honor it.

(A PRAYER FOR TODAY)

Thank you, God, for my body, this sacred temple that you've given me to grow, sustain, nourish, and birth life. May I meet my body with love and acceptance every single day.

A note on remembering

My meditation practice was a nonnegotiable for me before becoming a mother. I would wake up, and before even brushing my teeth, I would sit down to practice. It always felt like a download from God before starting the day. It fueled me. And then I became a mother and the days blurred together. I was tired. I lost my practice, pushing it to the side because it was the easiest thing to let go of.

One morning, I headed out of the house to grab a coffee and noticed a parked car outside my house with a bumper sticker that read *Discipline is a remembering of what you want most in this world.*

I always thought of discipline as negative or overly regimented, something I lacked when I was feeling lazy. But as a remembering? I had never heard it described in this way. I used this mindset as a way to start encouraging my morning meditation practice back into my daily routine, reminding myself that it was making me a more grounded, regulated mother for my baby.

Discipline is a commitment. It's a choice to show up over and over, despite what is going on around us. And each time we make that choice, we remember what is important. And we remember why.

What sets your heart on fire? What makes you feel alive? What makes you feel nourished? I know your baby means the world to you. As they should. But today, take some time to remember those things that are important to you outside of mothering your baby—those practices that help create the feelings that you want to cultivate, be it creativity or movement.

(A PRAYER FOR TODAY)

God, thank you for igniting my inner fire. As I embrace new passions, may I approach them with curiosity and openness.

Dream big, for both of you

I read something recently that said we would be foolish to love someone else's idea of motherhood because motherhood *is you*, it's who you need to be for your child. I have always loved to travel. It's one of the things that brought my partner and me together—our shared zest for adventure. And a part of me feared that seeing the world would stop once I was a mother, with the daily responsibilities of caring for my child. But did it have to? A few years ago, my partner and I began discussing a big trip we would take in the future, somewhere we've always wanted to go. And we did it. We packed up our little family and spent a month in Bali. It was everything I imagined it to be: salty hair, slow mornings, yoga and coffee, my son running around pointing at the monkeys and picking up the most peculiar insects in his hands to get a closer look. My second child on my hip. Your dreams start by speaking them out loud and by weaving them within your conversations with God.

So, I offer a gentle reminder to you today to let your own dreams unfurl alongside the ones you have for your child. You don't have to activate them immediately, but dreams provide hope and an energy that uplifts our spirits.

Your hopes for your baby's life and for your life get to coexist together. It's always both—and on this journey—not one or the other.

Sweet dreaming, Mama.

(A PRAYER FOR TODAY)

Today, I honor the dreams you have entrusted within me and the ones I have for my child. Let us be a portal of expansion for each other.

Reframe is the name of the game

In the whirlwind of motherhood, where the days often blur together and the to-do list seems endless, finding joy in the chaos can feel like a tall order. But here's the secret: it starts with a simple shift in perspective. I remember a moment when I was exhausted, overwhelmed, and feeling as though I was running on fumes. Then one day, I paused and realized I had been approaching everything from a place of obligation: *I have to feed him . . . I have to clean . . . I have to make dinner . . .*

But what if I changed the "I have to" to "I get to"?

I get to feed my baby, nourishing him.

I get to cook yummy meals for myself.

I get to nurture my body, honoring this vessel that carried new life.

I get to love my partner, deepening our bond.

I get to receive support, knowing I am not alone.

I get to be whoever I want to be.

The transformation was instant. It wasn't just about the words, it was the feeling behind them. There's a subtle but powerful shift in energy when we go from a sense of duty to a feeling of gratitude. This simple reframe uplifts the spirit and creates room for joy in everyday moments.

(A PRAYER FOR TODAY)

In each moment, I get to choose how I show up, how I respond, how I lead, how I love, who I choose to be.

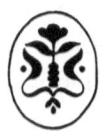

Sip of Self-Care:

Create a "joy jar." Find a jar, bowl, or container, and throughout the day, write down little moments of joy, anything that made you smile or feel grateful, no matter how small. It could be a beautiful sunset, a sweet nap with your baby, or a quiet cup of coffee. When you're feeling overwhelmed or need a boost, pull out a note from the jar and remember the goodness you've experienced. This practice helps you cultivate a habit of gratitude and brings moments of light into your day.

Sometimes subtraction is still additive

The life you are living right now, today, is said to be a product of the decisions you made three months ago. By this thinking, the decisions you are making right now will leave their mark on your future state three months from today. For this reason, every few months, I like to intentionally do a "life edit." In this exercise I not only look at the things, people, and experiences my soul longs to *bring in*, but I also look at what needs to go, what needs to be altered, and what parts of my life feel challenging and why.

It's easy to keep adding to our life, but when was the last time you subtracted something? Something that is weighing you down, sucking your energy; something that is siphoning more mental and physical energy than it deserves. By taking things off our plate and out of our life, we make room for what we want to cultivate to create a more balanced and authentic existence.

So, pay attention to what doesn't feel good. Ignorance tells us that if we simply ignore the heavy parts of our life, they go away. But they don't. They get louder and take up more space. And there is little value in holding on to what is no longer serving us.

You are the curator of your life. Cull things out until all that's left are the people and things you love.

(A PRAYER FOR TODAY)

God, allow me to decipher what is meant for me and what is not. Help me edit my life to live a deeper, more fulfilled and impactful life.

The firsts of many firsts

The firsts of many firsts—celebrate it all. You're experiencing and witnessing so many firsts together with your baby.

The first time they sleep for a longer stretch of time (maybe).

The first time they smile at the sound of your voice.

The first time they roll over onto their tummy and lift up their head.

The first time they say "Mama" or "Dada."

Their first holiday season.

Their first time meeting your family.

They might not remember it all, but there will be signs of how you celebrated during these milestones, in how you enveloped them in love. Their confidence and secure attachment reflect your care. So, document it if you feel called to—in your phone album, in a voice note, or in a baby journal you give to them when they're older.

Allow these moments to nourish you through this Winter season of deep transformation.

(A PRAYER FOR TODAY)

Thank you, God, for all the firsts with my baby. I am so grateful and honored to witness each of these milestones.

Eyes of wonder

Nourish your curiosity; it is the spark that keeps life vibrant and endlessly fascinating. Consider this: Your baby began as an egg within you, even before you were born. They've been a part of your life from the very start, and now they're before you, with their starry eyes and tender heart, a living testament to your shared journey.

Imagine if you could see the world through your baby's eyes—every moment experienced anew with wonder and delight. Feel the texture of each experience, listen to the symphony of new sounds, and embrace new perspectives and hobbies with a childlike eagerness. What if you approached each day as if it were a fresh adventure, each experience a discovery?

How exhilarating and refreshing would that be? As mothers, we are in a constant state of learning, and our little ones are powerful teachers guiding us on this path. What valuable lessons have they shared with you? Lean into those insights and let them enrich your life.

What stirs your curiosity? Explore that feeling with openness and joy, allowing God and life to surprise you in the most beautiful and unexpected ways.

(A PRAYER FOR TODAY)

Let me approach every experience with the heart of a child—curious, free, and uninhibited. And may I release all my preconceived notions. Keep my eyes of wonder open wide.

Give yourself space

Love needs room to grow. And so do you.

As you settle into your new routines and a new life with your baby, love needs freedom to explore. And so do you. To play and be curious. To find a new equilibrium, a new cadence so that you can thrive. In this serene pause, there is space for quiet growth and transformation. Just as winter's stillness allows nature to rest and renew, this season of motherhood is here to provide moments of deep reflection and nurturing, if you let it. Where do you need to give yourself the grace and space to create the fertile ground for the seasons ahead?

(A PRAYER FOR TODAY)

Let me lean into the spaciousness that this initiation of motherhood is asking of me.

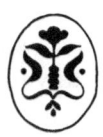

Sip of Self-Care:

Trataka Meditation

Light a candle and focus on the flame.

Allow your gaze to soften but remain intense and relaxed so that the flame shifts gently out of focus.

When your mind wanders, return to the flame.

Do this for three minutes and work your way up to five minutes.

Your inner landscape

The mechanical repetition of the "ch-ch-whoosh" sound of the breast pump will be forever etched in my mind. But as much as I didn't like being tethered to this device, I found myself appreciating the ten to fifteen minutes or so of being alone. It was a small window of opportunity to check in with myself, to take off my caretaker hat for just a few moments. Especially when I was feeling vulnerable and raw, emotional and sensitive to the energies surrounding me. There were many times my heart was heavy with the weight of loving my little one so much while trying to navigate our new environment.

How has the arrival of your little one transformed the landscape of your heart in this season of new motherhood? What are some emotions that surface as you continue to walk deeper into it?

As much as you may still feel like you're walking a bridge between two worlds (who you were before motherhood and who you are now), you are not lost. Here, within your newest initiation, you are found. You are evolving. You are becoming who you're meant to be, learning the new terrain of your inner world as you reconcile it with what is present in your outer world. Take a few moments to tend to her.

(A PRAYER FOR TODAY)

God, make room in my heart for all that is to come. Transform the landscape of my heart into a state of peace.

A spectrum

Over four months in and I still feel like I am trying to find my footing. The word "still" stings in my mind as I hear it. I can feel it in my bones—the disheartening and unmet expectation that I would have this all figured out by now. I am still stumbling over my own words, relearning my body and my baby. I'm still not sleeping. As I sobbed to my therapist, I described the details of my disappointment over not being able to pull it together in the way I used to. She listened with grace, then simply said, "Being human is a process."

And she's right. The problem wasn't the pace of my healing or the looming return to work. The real issue was that I hadn't allowed myself to be okay being in the gray space, the space where things are uncertain or unfinished. You see, we are always somewhere on the spectrum within different areas of our lives. Because being a human is a process, a journey—not a destination.

There is no healed version of you. We are always healing.

We never become. We are always becoming.

There is no perfect version. We are always evolving. We are always somewhere along the continuum.

And right now, in this moment, we need an unshakable trust in the higher power that is God, together with a healthy dose of surrender. Because sometimes, the greatest strength is not in having it all figured out but in having the courage to live in the unknown.

(A PRAYER FOR TODAY)

I pray for signs from you reassuring me I am meant to be in process. May your guidance and grace bring me peace in the uncertainties and may they illuminate the path ahead. Help me trust in your timing and wisdom as I navigate the journey of this life as a mother.

You were made to withstand the storms

Somewhere along the way in my life, I took on the role of problem solver for myself, for my family, and for those around me. As a lawyer, I could help people navigate the system. As an extrovert, I felt confident asking for things others didn't, and for a lot of my life, this served me well.

When it came to being a mother, things like sleeping, rashes, and teething were just other problems to solve. But I found the more books I devoured, the more blogs and online forums I searched, the more confused I felt. The information became a wind tunnel in my mind, and I didn't know which way was out.

I recently read that when it rains, a butterfly stops as quickly as possible. It seeks refuge under leaves, protecting its delicate wings from the pelting droplets by pressing them close to its body. And it waits, patiently and still, for the storm to pass. It sits in observation as the world around it transforms.

This is what I was missing—a quiet moment of retreat to let the storms of my mind settle. In the turbulence of sleepless nights and endless needs, I just needed to fold myself around my baby, creating a sanctuary of warmth and love. I needed to let the voice within carry the answers *to me* instead of the other way around.

Today, let each challenge serve as a gentle reminder of your boundless strength and tender vulnerability. And as the rain eventually subsides, the butterfly will emerge, renewed and vibrant, just as you will. You will find your rhythm and grace in the gentle dawning of each new day.

(A PRAYER FOR TODAY)

May I embody the lessons and evolution my baby's growth ignites in me.

You deserve grace as you find your footing

Childbirth and the postpartum months are two of the most profound, earth-shaking experiences a woman endures in her life. And here's the thing: you experience them back-to-back. So, give your emotions grace. Every day is different. You, too, are different.

Grace, from what I've experienced, is the art of accepting yourself, your circumstances, and those around you, as they are. With compassion. And with loving kindness. The definition of grace is offering "unmerited love." You don't have to earn it, it's a gift that you give just because you can. And in this tender season of your life, grace is something you can choose to offer yourself.

Your emotions in matrescence may feel like a wild roller coaster—sometimes you're high, other times low. What matters most is that you don't shame or judge yourself for feeling the way you do. Your emotions don't need fixing, they need understanding. They don't need suppression, they need exploration.

So, Mama, offer yourself the same compassion and kindness you so freely extend to others. Because grace isn't just about *enduring* these transformative moments—it's about *honoring* the beautiful, messy, and ever-changing journey of becoming.

(A PRAYER FOR TODAY)

May I extend love, compassion, and kindness to myself as I continue deepening my journey as a mother.

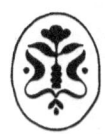

Sip of Self-Care:

Walk outside this morning, close your eyes, and let the sunlight wash over your face. Take three deep breaths and feel your feet being held from the ground up. Visualize the energy of the earth rising through your feet, flowing up your legs, filling your center, and spreading through your arms, throat, and crown, grounding you in the present moment.

Patience like a mother

Nobody understands patience quite like a mother. Patience is simply kindness in another form, a manifestation of love from a different vantage point. It involves holding your tongue, choosing your words carefully, and breathing through annoyance. You possess more capacity than you realize to embrace all these challenges, and that's the truth.

Your patience will be the most exercised muscle during the adventure of motherhood. I quickly learned that patience can wane even for those you adore on the deepest level, like your baby or your partner. However, the best lessons often emerge from moments that test our patience. Whether it's cleaning spit-up and a diaper explosion right after you've showered, or dealing with a well-meaning neighbor who stops by uninvited despite bringing meals and gifts, your patience is an endurance exercise. It strengthens your tolerance, acceptance, and compassion for the whole world as you know it.

I'm not suggesting you abandon boundaries or silence your voice when advocating for your needs. But on days that take unexpected detours, can you meet the moment with *softness*? Can you dig deep within yourself and choose kindness over frustration?

In the end, perhaps nothing truly matters on this earth except the love you give and the love you receive. So, in moments of impatience or when you feel like you're at your wits' end, take a deep breath.

You've got this. You have patience like a mother.

(A PRAYER FOR TODAY)

Teach me how to approach every situation with patience, acceptance, and openness. May I emulate the same love that you show to me every day, without judgment or limitation.

Power and possibility

When I first became a mother, someone told me, "You're shaping the future with every small thing you do." I remember laughing nervously—how could that be true when I felt like I was just trying to survive sleepless nights and endless diaper changes? But one day, while rocking my baby to sleep, it hit me: this little life in my arms was looking to me to teach him not only how to walk but how to navigate the world.

Mothers are powerful, and while it might sound like a cliché, it's the absolute truth. You possess the remarkable ability to shape not just the present but also future generations through your voice, your words, your thoughts, and your actions in mothering.

I know this responsibility can feel immense. I've felt it too. The leaders of tomorrow are nurtured and guided within our homes today. You have the profound potential to transform the parenting paradigm, to forge new paths and create new ways of being. But here's what I've learned: you don't have to do it perfectly. Your choices—every "yes" and every "no"—carry a sacred power when you honor the truth they reveal and the guidance they provide.

This role isn't just about responsibility, it's about *possibility*. By mothering with intention and heart, you become a figure of transformation in your lineage—a woman who dared to create new ways of being, forging a path of love and purpose for those who come after her.

The way you mother today will weave a story that lasts far beyond your lifetime. That's your power. That's your legacy. And it's extraordinary.

(A PRAYER FOR TODAY)

Thank you for giving me this power and responsibility of being a mother. May I revere it and harness it in a way that feels aligned for me, my baby, and my family.

Embrace your body in all her glory and shifts

I trust that I'm in a season of rebuilding, gently restoring my strength and stamina. I am nourishing my postpartum hormones, giving my body the time and space it needs to recalibrate.

In this journey, I'm discovering the beauty in my scars—whether physical or emotional—and learning to honor my stretch marks and the new capacities of my body. This is a time for me to love my body in all her transformations, celebrating her strength, resilience, and the way she's forever changed. It's easy to be influenced by what others, or the media, suggest is the "right" time to redefine or heal, but I know that only I can decide my own pace.

And so, Mama, remember this for yourself too. Listen closely to what your body is telling you. Hold her with love in this tender and powerful moment. Your body is capable of incredible magic and strength—just like mine—as she created, carried, nourished, and brought a new life into the world. Embrace your body in all her glory; offer her the credit she deserves.

(A PRAYER FOR TODAY)

Thank you for this powerful vessel. May I always treat her with love, kindness, and compassion.

Trust fall into motherhood

Have you ever had those moments when you doubt every decision you're making for your baby?

I remember the first time my baby had a cold. My family was in town. He was feverish, aching, and crying nonstop. I tried everything I could think of—herbal remedies, a warm bath, bouncing, distraction tactics: basically all the tricks I knew—but nothing seemed to help. I just couldn't figure out why he wouldn't stop crying. It was heartbreaking. Eventually, both of us were exhausted, and we retreated to the back bedroom. I wrapped a blanket around his back and laid him on my chest for in skin-to-skin contact. He then settled and nursed. In that quiet moment, it hit me—this was what he'd needed all along, alone time with me. I realized he could sense my emotions and was overwhelmed by them.

It was in that stillness that I learned to trust my own authority, my power, and I learned to assert myself patiently, kindly, and compassionately. I told my self-doubt: "I am new at this and that's all right. You can take a step back, with love. I won't let you steal my peace or my confidence or my innate wisdom I have to be a mother to my baby."

Self-doubt does not define who we are as a mother. Doubt simply means that we are still learning. Here we are, a little over four months in, finding our way through this beautiful, messy journey of motherhood.

(A PRAYER FOR TODAY)

In moments when I doubt myself, may I be reminded that doubt is only here as a spectator, not a copilot. May I remember to give myself grace, compassion, and love.

Sip of Self-Care:

The Bowl of Clarity

Write down your worries on small slips of paper and place them in a bowl. Light a candle and hold the bowl in your hands. Whisper: "These concerns are not bigger than my ability to grow and learn." As you burn the slips one by one in a safe, fireproof container, imagine each worry transforming into light, clearing space for your inner wisdom to shine through.

Grief and gratitude: two things can be true

It's okay to grieve who you were as you embrace who you're becoming, Mama. Two truths can coexist. Maternal mentor, educator, and author Jessie Harrold reminds us that you can't grow without grief. In her book *Mothershift*[9], she explains that grief has four needs: to be felt, honored, metabolized, and sometimes, released.

Motherhood isn't for the faint of heart. It's a journey full of contradictions. I felt galvanized by the idea of returning to my work in philanthropy while feeling heartbroken about missing time with my baby. This was new for me—the feeling of opposite emotions living side by side, chasing my mind like a tug-of-war between light and shadow. Both pulled me in different directions as I searched for my footing in this new terrain.

There will be days when you long for the version of you who moved freely, unbound by feeding schedules, nap times, and diaper changes. Yet, in the same moment, you'll feel a surge of gratitude for exactly where you are: snuggling your sweet baby, breathing in their scent, kissing their toes endlessly, and connecting with them on the deepest level.

There will be days when you grieve the woman you once were. And yet, you will also feel a fierce love for the woman you are now: the one who chooses to carry a baby on her hip, who is learning that rest is a form of resilience, and who is beginning to shed the societal expectations of being a "boss babe" or "supermom."

If today your heart feels tender with old memories as you navigate this unfolding identity, know that it's okay. It's normal to grieve as you let go and reinvent yourself. Grief doesn't mean you're broken; it means you're growing.

Just remember that who you're becoming and where you're going is far more abundant than where you've ever been.

(A PRAYER FOR TODAY)

Let me find reverence for who I have been and who I am becoming. Both get to coexist. I know and trust a whole new version of who I am meant to be is being born.

Bend so you don't break

There was a moment when I knew my son was tired. I had already nursed him three times within an hour, and yet he would wake as soon as I laid him down. I could feel my level of patience waning, my peace unearthed, as I sat back in the rocking chair to try once more to get him to sleep. I hadn't eaten dinner. My back was sore, and my body ached. My partner popped his head in the room and asked if he could try. I felt the hesitation well up in my body.

I am the mother. I should have endless patience. I should be able to do this. What kind of mother am I if I need a break from my baby?

But this kind of self-talk does not serve anyone. I know this now. For I am human, a being who needs to recharge and refuel just like any other person. And it's all about perspective. It's not a break from my baby, it's an opportunity to reset. Endless patience is not required when you have endless love. We are all doing our best in every moment.

But you are adaptable and that requires you to sometimes go with the flow, to be flexible, to be resilient, and to stay open to what the moment *is* versus what you want it to be.

Sounds a lot like motherhood, doesn't it?

Since that day there have been many times I have (after making sure my baby is safe) walked away for two minutes to collect myself, allowed my partner to tap in, or given myself permission to cry alongside my baby in the heat of a hard moment.

Remember this the next time you're doubting yourself: You are the mother God chose for your baby. Your decision to bend your own rules can sometimes be the greatest show of strength.

Bend, Mama, so you don't break.

(A PRAYER FOR TODAY)

Dear God, guide me to move in alignment with your direction and flow for me and my baby. May I be open to receiving the support you have surrounded me with and remind me often that this motherhood journey does not have to look a certain way. Help me to embrace change with an open heart, to learn from challenges, and to flourish in the face of uncertainty.

Be careful what you wish for

I know it's easy to wish you were already past the waves you may be experiencing right now in motherhood—the teething, the witching hour, the gassy days (and nights), the sick days . . . all of them.

However, wishing them away isn't going to speed up the process. The time will pass anyway, whether you are present or zoning out. I often remind myself that God didn't create a fast-forward button on our lives for a reason. Neither did he create a pause button. Marinate on this for a moment: We will never get this time again and we don't have the power to stop time. I'm not saying you have to enjoy every moment, but try to be there for it nonetheless, knowing that it won't last forever (thankfully).

These hard days may even be the memories you fondly look back on and reminisce about later on in life. My mother still likes to tell the story of how I woke her up at 3 a.m., bright eyed and bushy tailed, for months on end. She laughs when she thinks back to those wee hours of the night when it was just the two of us. But her eyes also get teary as she recounts the experience because while they were hardest at times, they were also bittersweet.

So, don't wish away the present moment, Mama. Instead, bring yourself back by focusing on your baby's tiny hands and little lips. Every moment matters, for you, your baby, and your family. You're creating memories of a lifetime.

(A PRAYER FOR TODAY)

May I be ever present in the moments of my life and my baby's life. May I be mindful and intentional about how I show up and how I devote my time and energy to all of us.

Savor the partnership, Mama

I know it might feel like you and your partner are like ships passing in the night, especially in this early season of motherhood. But savor the in-between moments with each other. Leave each other cute notes. Don't stop connecting in each other's love languages just because you are now learning to integrate parenthood into your lives.

Be intentional about carving out even a few minutes, or if you can, an hour, when you sit with each other and talk about something other than the baby.

Something I heard recently from a relationship therapist is the 7-7-7 rule to help your partnership thrive. In the 7-7-7 rule, every 7 days you head out to dinner or a coffee date, or explore something new together, without your baby. Every 7 weeks, you take an overnight trip together. And every 7 months, you go away for weekend (or longer vacation) together as a couple.

If the above doesn't work for you or your family's needs, don't worry. Find a cadence that does work. What matters most is that you continue to prioritize each other and don't lose sight of one another along the way as you walk this journey of parenthood together.

(A PRAYER FOR TODAY)

God, thank you for our relationship and the beautiful family we are growing together. Thank you for the support, love, nourishment, and expansion I receive from my partner daily.

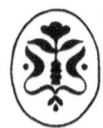

Sip of Self-Care:

Spend some time pondering and talking to your partner about a regular routine of spending time together. While this may seem overly architected, it is often necessary in the whirlwind of this period. Maybe one of the 7-7-7 rules works for you (which are more of a fun guideline), or maybe something else feels right. Make it your own, make it intentional, and notice how you feel when you have watered the relationship with your partner. If you are uncoupled, do this same exercise with a friend or someone you value greatly in your life.

Let kind candor lead your way

There's wisdom in the old saying "honesty is the best policy," especially when paired with kindness and compassion. On this journey of motherhood, almost five months in, you've likely encountered a flood of unsolicited advice—dos and don'ts, parenting tips, and partner guidance. It's enough to make anyone's head spin, especially when you're still learning to find your rhythm.

Here's where the power of your throat chakra comes in. Chakras are considered energy centers in the body that govern different aspects of our physical, emotional, and spiritual well-being. The throat chakra, located in the center of your neck, represents your ability to communicate your truth with clarity, kindness, and authenticity. When it's balanced, you can express yourself with confidence and compassion, setting boundaries that honor both you and others.

For example, when faced with advice that doesn't align with your path, you might gently say, "Thank you for your guidance, but I am learning to find my own groove as a mother." This kind of honesty doesn't require anger or defensiveness—it's simply your truth, spoken with grace.

Whatever your path, you can set boundaries with kindness. Stay sovereign in an unsound world by letting kindness lead the way with radical candor. Those who understand will support you, and those who don't respect it—bless and release them without making a big deal. Embrace your journey with confidence, knowing that your truth, shared with grace, is your strength and your sanctuary.

(A PRAYER FOR TODAY)

It is safe to speak my truth. It is safe to uphold my boundaries. It is safe to advocate for my needs and what is best for me and my baby.

The yin and yang of motherhood

Brené Brown wittingly pointed out that it's "[o]nly when we are brave enough to explore the darkness will we discover the infinite power of our light."[10] You see, it's the contrasts are what make each moment beautiful.

Light and dark.

Joy and sadness.

Calm and chaos.

Peace and restlessness.

Late nights and early mornings.

Blissful moments followed by moments of meltdowns.

The plot twists you didn't see coming.

Contrasts in your motherhood are what make it stand out. They're what make it all worthwhile.

Life would be dull if you didn't have the shenanigans, antics, cute moments, nerve-racking moments, the highs and lows there to give you variety, experience, and wisdom. Let the contrast create the intricate design of your unique story.

(A PRAYER FOR TODAY)

Teach me to walk, dance, relish, and appreciate the daily contrasts of my life and motherhood.

You are the butterfly

Today, I could feel myself morphing in small ways. Some of my thought patterns still feel foreign, and my priorities are shifting. As grateful as I am to be a mother, I also have moments of uncertainty about how I want my life to look going forward.

I read a story about a butterfly and its process. We know the caterpillar turns into a butterfly, but it's the in-between that we don't really think about. The caterpillar dissolves in the cocoon then reconfigures itself and its molecules completely. Does it know what is waiting on the other side? Or does it just trust the process?

The in-between is not always pretty. For the caterpillar, it literally becomes a mushy goo with no semblance of its prior self except for tiny imaginal discs that carry forward its memories/learnings from its previous form. Because all rebirth requires transformation, a death or falling away of parts of our old self must occur to make room for the new. And that's where I feel I am right now, and maybe you feel that way too.

So, let me be the first to remind you, Mama. You are the butterfly. Even if right now, you are living in the mushy goo.

(A PRAYER FOR TODAY)

God, thank you for this gift of life and motherhood. Help me embrace the transformation this season brings as I rise from the ashes, leaning into the greatest initiation of my life.

Your words matter

Our words matter—I've always known that—especially in relationships. But to a growing, forming brain, they mean everything. We decipher our baby's special code (crying, body movements, smiles, hand gestures) and turn it into language. Our baby looks to us to describe everything from people to feelings, and they pick up on it all. Therefore, I invite you to bring intention into the script for reading all the messages of this little somatic being.

A therapist friend of mine mentioned that she has patients who are still grappling with the labels their parents put on them as a child. Perhaps, then, we should be clear with ourselves about why we choose one word over another. How does the word make you feel when you say it? For me, a word that always irks me is "fussy" because it typically has negative connotations. When my baby cries, for example, people ask me if he is *being* fussy, thus insinuating that he isn't behaving. Our babies cry to communicate! So, I've started using the word "fizzy" instead, and it feels much more neutral, less loaded. Fizzy means that my baby is letting out energy. It hasn't taken long for others in my orbit caring for my baby to start using the term, as have my friends. It's a small change, but it has a ripple effect on the way we'll remember things.

Did I have a fussy baby? Nope, just a bit of fizz from time to time.

(A PRAYER FOR TODAY)

God, help me speak the words that ring true and offer grace and kindness for my baby and me. Let these words be like healing balm, offering a gentleness to every situation we encounter.

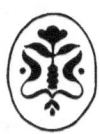

Sip of Self-Care:

Words shape our energy. Take a moment to reflect on the language you use with yourself and your baby. Choose a few phrases to gently swap:

- Instead of "I'm so tired," try "I'm giving myself grace today."
- Instead of "Why are you so sad," try "You're sharing your feelings with me."

Write down these swaps and place them somewhere visible. Throughout the day, pause and practice replacing old words with these softer, more loving alternatives. Small shifts in language create big shifts in energy—for you and your baby.

The wonderful world of word swaps

Building on yesterday's entry, here are a few other "word swaps" I have found supportive. They may seem subtle, but I invite you to "try them on" and see how they feel in your body, mind, and home.

Breakthrough vs. *tantrum/meltdown*

Maybe your child hasn't had one of these yet, but they will, eventually. Terms like "meltdown" and "tantrum" signal that there has been a malfunction or some ill intent. Instead, a positive word swap is "emotional release" or "emotional expression." My favorite is "breakthrough" because you have to have a breakdown to break through, right? These alternatives reiterate a child expressing their feelings in a healthy, natural, and very developmentally appropriate way.

Sleep progression vs. *regression*

Your baby is always moving forward. Period. They are learning, evolving, and growing at an extremely rapid rate. Instead of framing it as a setback or regression, "sleep progression" highlights the forward movement and evolution of a child's sleep habits even if they are temporarily sleeping less. This term encourages us to view our child's sleep changes as opportunities for learning and adaption rather than sources of frustration or concern. It promotes a positive mindset and helps us approach sleep challenges with patience, understanding, and optimism.

I encourage you to build upon this list and to notice the words that you, and other caretakers around your child, use on a regular basis.

(A PRAYER FOR TODAY)

God, allow me to set the stage for my baby to feel empowered by my words, as these words will eventually flow from their lips as well. May I marinate on certain terms in my heart and know whether they are right for my family.

Every beginning comes from some other beginning's end

Fed is best, Mama. We are always doing the best we can in every moment so know that your choices are made with love and are therefore valid. Always.

However you choose to feed your baby, be it breast, formula, or donor breast milk, know that it's your choice. Don't let anyone shame you into thinking otherwise. We are all doing the best we can, and we love our babies with every ounce of our being. I know that, and you know that. At some point your breastfeeding journey will come to an end. By this time in my journey, I was having severe dips in my supply and was so afraid of an "ending." It was emotional and heavy. We managed to find our way through for a few more months, but in looking back, had our journey ended at that point, it would have led to the beginning of another chapter for my baby and me.

Every circumstance is multifactorial, and stress plays a crucial role in your milk supply. So, wherever you find yourself, trust your body, trust your baby's cues, and lean into this knowing that as long as they are fed and nourished, they will grow to thrive.

(A PRAYER FOR TODAY)

My baby is always nourished through me, with me. May I remember that as long as they are nourished, healthy, and safe, that is all that matters. God, help me attune to the needs and voice of my body and baby and drown out the noise of others' opinions.

It's okay to cry

If it makes you cry, it's because it matters to you. It doesn't make you weak, it makes you human. Things that don't matter to you don't have the power to awaken your tear ducts. Tears of joy, tears of sadness, tears of anger and overwhelm, even tears for seemingly no reason at all signify that you are feeling *something*.

Did you know that humans produce three types of tears—basal, reflex, and emotional? Our body is so wise, and each type of tear has a unique purpose. Basal tears are the ones we don't notice; they constantly lubricate our eyes to keep them moist and healthy and even contain enzymes to help fight infections. Reflex tears happen when something irritates our eyes—like onions, smoke, or dust—and help wash away those irritants. And then there are emotional tears, which occur in response to strong feelings like joy, sadness, or frustration. These tears contain higher levels of stress hormones and proteins, suggesting that when released, they may play a role in reducing stress or processing emotions. Moreover, emotional crying can have a healing effect as well. Crying releases endorphins, natural painkillers, which may explain why people often feel a sense of relief or catharsis after a good cry.

So, give yourself permission to cry it out, shake it out, and shed everything that comes up for release. Let it all be a sign for how much you care—reframe it as a way to get rid of pent-up tension or stress in your body.

Feel to heal it.

(A PRAYER FOR TODAY)

God, let me see the lessons, the release, and the blessings in each tear I shed. May I recognize that expressing my emotions is a sign of strength and not a weakness.

You hold the paintbrush

This is your time to create the design of your motherhood experience.

Perhaps there were certain moments growing up when you wished your parents did things differently (even if they did the best with what they knew and had at the time). Guess what? You get to implement those shifts now.

Create what you desire in terms of family lifestyle, work–life balance, and relationships you envision in life. It all starts and ends with you, Mama. You are the visionary, the author of your motherhood journey. It's not about being perfect, it's about being unique and true to yourself.

(A PRAYER FOR TODAY)

God, bless the visions you've given me and guide me to birth them in alignment with my highest self and the highest, most benevolent good of all.

Sip of Self-Care:

Place your hand over your heart and repeat: "There is no greater mother for my baby than me."

If you have time today, break out the watercolors and let yourself paint freely.

Shedding what no longer serves you

What are you shedding right now? Whatever it is, let it fall away.

Habits that once felt second nature may not fit you anymore. Friendships that once felt good may no longer feel aligned because they either don't understand or respect your journey, or perhaps you've outgrown the relationship. Family relationships take on a new tone and nuance, and sometimes distance and boundaries make for good relations. You're not as available as you once were—for counsel, input, or any other form of resourcefulness—because you are needed for yourself, your baby, and the new family you're growing.

What are you being asked to shed? Let it fall away gracefully. It doesn't need to be a big scene or a hard conversation (although sometimes these are necessary). It only needs you to unplug your energy supply from it.

Like a snake shedding its skin, release what you've outgrown so you can continue to expand.

Remember, where your focus goes, your energy flows. Where your energy flows, you grow.

(A PRAYER FOR TODAY)

Help me release everything that no longer nourishes me. It's the most selfless act of love I could ever give to myself and my baby.

A moving prayer

I picked up the phone today as I sat rocking my son. It was my sister-in-law, and she was calling to tell me her big news: She was going on a ten-day silent retreat. We had both taken the same meditation teacher training and were passionate about mindfulness and slow living. *Wow*, I thought. *Ten days? In silence?* I tried to listen to her talk, but a wave of emotion rose within my chest, filling it quickly until it was on the brink of a cascade.

It was the first time I've had this feeling or, rather, the realization that there are limits to the things I can do now that I am a mother. Before motherhood, I would have been able to consider attending this retreat and plan my life accordingly to make it happen. But now? There is no way. I can barely take a few hours away from my baby. Right now, I am so needed in this chapter, I can't even imagine a future date for when I will be able to embrace this type of experience. It feels heavy, like a loss.

As I sat with my reaction for the remainder of today, I questioned why this ignited something within me. Did I want to go on the retreat? No, but I did want the space to go deeper, to reach a new level of inspiration. So, I decided to commit to offering myself a half-day mini silent retreat. I would be silent in my own home.

Today, I invite you to give yourself the gift of silent observation, of silent moving meditation. Even for an hour.

Easier said than done? I know. But breathe into it. Feel into it.

(A PRAYER FOR TODAY)

May I listen to the answers of my soul in these moments of peace and quiet. May I choose to break silence with intentional words rooted in love.

The surrender experiment

We all want to "get it right" (whatever that means to you). But the truth is, so much of motherhood requires experimentation. What works? What doesn't? And it's not a "one and done" experiment. It involves trying things over and over, some of which will flop while others land. If I feed a bit longer, will he sleep better? If I play this song when he is in the car seat, will it make for a more enjoyable ride for all of us (especially my nervous system)? My baby didn't like the swing last week, but maybe this week will be different—let's give it a whirl?

The only difference between an expert and a novice (or a seasoned mom and a new one) is that the former has experimented more times. They've had more chances to learn. To refine our mothering, we just have to try and be okay with the times it doesn't work out. Those are valuable experiments too.

How would it feel to see your day as little experiments? Just good old trial and error? How would it feel to release the expectation of getting it right? To move past the fear of a wrong turn? To find freedom in simply choosing a different way the next time if it didn't work out as you wanted?

All good things have come from someone's experiment. So, take the pressure off, Mama. Surrender to the flow of simply trying something with a dollop of curiosity.

(A PRAYER FOR TODAY)

God, may I embrace the freedom to experiment, trusting that your wisdom will guide me in every step. Let my heart remain open to new ideas and approaches, finding joy in the adventure of nurturing my child.

You don't have to be the person you have always been

It's time for reinvention, recalibration, reorganization, reorientation.

Who are you called to be? I know, it's a brand-new identity you've taken on—Mama, Mom, Mother.

You're in that liminal space right now where you walk the fine line of embracing who you were as you step into who you are called to be.

What does this new version of you love?

What does she no longer tolerate?

What does she allow into her life?

Who does she remove from her life?

How does she move? How does she lead?

You are reinventing yourself and shedding everything that no longer fits your evolution.

(A PRAYER FOR TODAY)

Guide me to be who you are calling me to be in this season of my life, without apology, without guilt, without any inhibitions.

Sip of Self-Care:

Journal on the questions from Day 144 and spend a few minutes
praying over them, inviting God to bring these visions to life.

The famous mama two-step

Motherhood is a sacred dance that you will master and refine over a whole lifetime. And when you look back on these moments, you will beam with love, pride, joy, and so much soul.

Somedays this dance is exhilarating; you're learning new steps, new routines, new cadences (yours and your baby's)—you're confidently and boldly taking a step forward. The same may be true with your relationship with your partner—as parents, as companions, as soul carriers of this beautiful life you have birthed.

Somedays this dance is exhausting. You wonder whether it will ever end. It feels like there is always a fire to put out, a mountain to climb. Or perhaps you're dealing with other heaviness in your life or your baby's. In these moments, it may feel like you are taking steps backward. But there is still movement nonetheless. There is a pace, and when you zoom out, there is a harmonious flow to the path you are exploring.

So dance. Find your own cadence, your own groove, your own rhythm so you can move to the heartbeat of your soul.

(A PRAYER FOR TODAY)

Dear God, teach me how to dance with the upswings and downswings—the beautiful cadence of motherhood with which I've been blessed.

Abundance is a frequency that you are attuned to

Nurture the abundance in your life, Mama. New life, new birth, new you, new baby, new routines. All of it is abundant.

There is an abundance of time, even if it feels scarce. This is when presence comes into play—the slower you move, the longer and richer time will feel. There is an abundance of resources. Some may be more tangible than others but don't forget about the deep well of strength and wisdom within you. On days when it feels like resources are scarce (which they can be depending on circumstances), tap into your body and notice the abundance it holds, creates, nourishes, and sustains. You birthed your baby! Notice your breath; notice your heart beating. You are alive and safe. Notice the roof over your head, the warm bed you sleep in, the clothes you have to wear, the food you are able to eat, the simple luxuries you're able to afford, and the necessities you have. Notice the abundance of love and friendship and connection in your life.

Abundance is all around us—we just need to take a moment to witness it and express gratitude for it. It is a frequency that we can attune ourselves to if we want.

You are abundance personified.

(A PRAYER FOR TODAY)

Thank you, God, for all the abundance in my life that nourishes me and my baby.

The triage rule

Practice the triage rule.

A dear friend shared this powerful concept with me one day when I was overwhelmed. She was already a few years into motherhood and had multiple children. Who better to ask for counsel and advice than her, a trusted friend, a seasoned mama?

As I shared and vented about my day, she asked me a few questions:

- "What matters the most right now?"
- "Out of everything on your plate, what are three things you absolutely need to do today? Focus only on those for today."
- "And what are three things you need to do this week, nonnegotiably?"

She called this the triaging method. Much like how the ER at the hospital triages patients and situations, motherhood will require you to triage daily. Not everything that feels urgent truly is. My husband, in his usual lighthearted way, often responds with a question when I ask for his help: "Is this a *now* thing?" At first, I'd roll my eyes or giggle, but now I've come to appreciate the question. Not everything needs immediate action. Some things can wait, and there's peace in recognizing that. Check in with your body, with your heart, and with your capacity. What do you most need in each moment, each day? Focus on those things.

(A PRAYER FOR TODAY)

In every situation, may I discern between what is required of me right now and what can wait until tomorrow. Rushing is not in my highest good.

*May you choose environments that bring out the softness
in you rather than the survival*

You define what makes you feel content, at peace.

You define the pace of your day, the types of rituals you engage in for yourself and your baby.

You create your own rulebook.

You can choose the environment that brings you peace—this includes behaviors, friendships and relationships, career choices, parenting styles, and everything in between.

During this season of motherhood, I had a friendship I found challenging. One thing that came out of me as we worked through our issues was this: I am a kind person, but that doesn't mean I am a *weak* person.

I can say no. I can have boundaries. I can remove myself from situations as needed.

It is a privilege to be in your orbit, so if there are people who are not treating that orbit with respect and kindness, then their chapter in your story may have run its course.

You get to define what a joyful, nourished motherhood looks and feels like to you. And I hope that you surround yourself with people that create an environment that brings out the softest version of you.

(A PRAYER FOR TODAY)

Help me choose peace above all. Help me fill my life with those that love and respect my baby and me.

Sip of Self-Care:

Begin to notice any negative physical reactions you have to certain people, conversations, places, and even entertainment (movies, TV shows) and learn from them. Do you feel overstimulated? Overwhelmed? Defensive? Check in with how you feel after interactions with certain people or experiences and then, if needed, limit or avoid inviting those people, thoughts, feelings, or experiences into your environment in the future.

Eyes open, mind open, heart open

This week one of my close friends (who doesn't have children yet) asked me to go to brunch. She said we could go to any of our usual favorite spots, but she was hoping to go before the restaurants filled up for the football game. She mentioned that we could even stay for the game . . .

My stomach dropped. Brunch? At a certain time? I am still figuring out so much of our routine. Also, I didn't want to be anywhere loud, and a football game was not on my list of desired activities. I could hear my inner dialogue, and I knew it sounded so different from my pre-baby self. I was tempted to say yes, but this latest version of me just wanted to make eggs and toast, cuddle up with a good matcha, and chat at home. I pondered what was wrong with me.

The answer? Nothing. So much of my experience these days is just new. I have never experienced these preferences, reactions, and feelings. I am in the portal of transformation, and everything feels like unchartered territory. Because it is. Do you feel it?

The most important thing we can do during these moments, however, is to stay open to the new, and not just the fact that you're new to motherhood, but all that this initiation brings. Stay open to loving a new way, moving a new way, speaking and communicating a new way. Stay open to new connections, different conversations, and an unchartered direction for your life and motherhood. You were chosen for this initiation. Remember that every initiation requires us to embrace new textures, new tastes, new rhythms, and new ways of being.

Stay open to your shifting form, for the more we learn about her now, in our Winter season, the more equipped we will be come Spring to plant the most fruitful seeds in the seasons ahead.

(A PRAYER FOR TODAY)

God, thank you for the gift of newness in my life through my motherhood. May I walk without judgment as I embark on this new chapter of self-discovery.

Your story creates your strength

Relish in your strength, Mama.

Just as a single snowflake might seem delicate and insignificant, when it joins countless others, it transforms into a mighty force. Together, these snowflakes cover large swaths of the land in a peaceful, unified blanket, defining the landscape with their presence. Your seemingly small, isolated choices weave together to create the story of your strength, just like these snowflakes.

Strength manifests differently each day. Some days it's found in allowing yourself to shed tears without hesitation. Other days it's in fully embracing laughter, savoring every moment without guilt or self-judgment. Strength can also be seen in taking a breath before responding impulsively or letting emotions dictate your actions. At times, it's about standing up for yourself and your baby with unwavering love and firmness. And sometimes strength means stepping away from toxic situations or people and prioritizing yourself and your baby over the demands of others.

We often search for God in places *other* than our own hearts, our own stories. So, remember, wherever you are, you don't need to search for strength—it will find you. It's already within you, ready to be accessed when you need it most.

Today, celebrate the many dimensions of your strength.

(A PRAYER FOR TODAY)

Thank you, God, for gracing me with strength to navigate each moment in my motherhood.

The door of creation

Some may think it's just the period of months that a baby inhabits a mother's body, but it's much deeper than that. In fact, your baby's DNA lives in your blood for years after birth, and some of their cells remain inside your tissue and brain for your entire life. This phenomenon is called fetal-maternal chimerism. Meaning, the creation of life in your womb is an invitation to be forever changed. From that moment on, your baby is a part of you on a cellular level. Mother and child, connected for eternity.

So, in those moments that feel dark and difficult now, remember that this is just the door of creation creaking ajar, letting light peek through, offering a glimpse of who you can be and who you are becoming—the mother born anew from what can feel like a fiery hull or the darkest of nights.

Like the phoenix rising from the ashes, you emerge bold and beautiful.

The door of creation has opened, inviting you to walk through. Remember that God and your baby didn't just choose you for who you are today but for the woman you are becoming as well.

(A PRAYER FOR TODAY)

Guide me to stand in my truth every day. Guide my words, my voice, my heart. It is safe to ask for what I need.

You are your baby's earth

Do you feel it, Mama? How your body, your presence, is their everything? You are their ground, their steady, unshakable earth. They sleep best on your chest because it feels like coming home. They reach for your arms because they know they'll find safety there. Skin to skin isn't just comfort, it's connection. It's their way of saying, "You are my world."

You are the river, nourishing them with milk.

You are the tree, standing tall, weathering storms, offering your branches for shelter and stability.

You are the breeze, your voice and touch calming them in their wildest cries.

You are the soil, rich with experiences, full of wisdom and patience that they can draw from.

You, Mama, are their earth. Their entire world, their source of life, much like earth sustains all living beings.

When they feed, it's from your body. When they cry, it's your warmth they seek. When they land—on your lap or against your heart—it's the softest, safest place they'll ever know. You matter more than you think. More than you may ever know.

Today, remember that you are your baby's earth.

(A PRAYER FOR TODAY)

God, provide me the grace to be a soft place for my baby to land, a gentle sanctuary of love and comfort. May my arms be a refuge of warmth and safety, my heart a wellspring of tenderness and understanding. Help me nurture and support my child with patience, kindness, and unwavering love, guiding them through life's journey with ongoing strength and deep compassion.

Sip of Self-Care:

Invite Joy In

Find a quiet space, take a deep breath, then say the following mantra aloud three times, slowly and intentionally:

"Joy is here."

As you speak, notice how the words land in your body. Feel their vibration settle into your chest, your heart, and your mind. Let each repetition remind you that joy isn't something to chase—it's already within you, waiting to be noticed.

Pause for a moment after the last repetition and let the simplicity of this truth fill you. Joy is here, and so are you.

The effortlessness of being

There is joy to be found in surrendering to the moment and allowing your day to unfold before you. Babies show us how to be perfectly present. They feel their emotions from moment to moment; as soon as the emotion arises and is felt, it leaves them. There is no trying to conceal it, hide it away, or bottle it up—your baby is a vessel for which "being" flows.

During this season, you are most likely seeing facets of your baby's personality and demeanor arise as they express themselves more. Maybe they are sleeping longer stretches or feeding less, or maybe you're waiting for these changes. But waiting and wanting interrupts *being*.

It takes so much energy and effort to constantly be striving, researching, worrying, planning, contemplating . . . and it's exhausting. Letting go of the need to control puts those resources back in your proverbial bank so you can build a reserve for these winter months.

So today, can you just be? If everything is great, be great. If things aren't, then that's okay too.

Your baby will only be this little in this moment, and you will only be this version of yourself right now. Don't let the worries of tomorrow steal the joy of today.

(A PRAYER FOR TODAY)

God, let me recognize the inherent value in the very existence of both my baby and myself.

Kindness as a healing salve

We were out of oatmeal (my morning go-to because it's quick and I can make it with one hand). And it was raining. The grocery store is only a three-minute walk around the corner, so I grabbed the umbrella, strapped my baby into the carrier against my chest, and stepped outside into the drizzly haze.

While in the store, I remembered a few more items we needed: milk, apples, and almond butter. I got in line and smiled at the cashier who looked back in annoyance as she dumped everything into a paper bag. *Ah, she must be having a bad day*, I thought.

As I reached the door to leave, it was now pouring. I covered us up and looked to make sure it was clear to cross the street. Water was pelting from every direction when I felt it—the bottom of the bag giving out. I heard my groceries splash across the sidewalk, and I became flustered and stressed. I checked to make sure that my baby was okay—yep, still sleeping (how was that possible?).

When I looked up, a woman was collecting my groceries in her arms. She offered to walk me home, and while I wanted to tell her that I had everything under control, I didn't. Tears stung the back of my eyes and felt salty in my throat.

The woman just smiled and said, "Hey, we are all in this together, right?"

Kindness is medicine. You never know how your actions will affect others. In moments when you want to say something snarky (because life happens and the days can get exhausting), pause, breathe, then step back into whatever it is you were doing with a more genuine tone. And in moments when it feels easier to shut down and numb out (because postpartum is heavy, and sometimes asking for support feels hard), ask yourself what you would do if you had a friend struggling in the same way. Give yourself permission to ask for the help you need.

Kindness will heal you inside and out. It will heal your relationship with your body, your mind, your abilities, your soul, your loved ones. But only if you lead from it.

(A PRAYER FOR TODAY)

May I be a channel of kindness and compassion.

Spring comes after the storm

You are built in the storms.

The strongest, deepest part of your soul is forged with strength from God.

The storms are not here to shake and uproot you. They're here to help uproot the people, places, and circumstances you have outgrown as you step into your next evolution and expansion.

The storms are here to rebuild you. You will come out the other side stronger, clearer, and more anchored in who you are meant to be.

Today, wherever you are, wherever you find yourself, know that every storm passes, and spring is around the corner. And right now, you are being refined, you are being anchored into your identity as a mother, the matriarch of your family.

Let the storms take their course; they will pass. Eventually, all storms run out of rain. Stay rooted in who you are at a soul level.

(A PRAYER FOR TODAY)

God, I know you walk with me in the storms of my life. Guide me, refine me, strengthen me on this journey of motherhood. Help me find the rainbow and the light in each moment of heaviness.

A perfectly imperfect life

The moments we experience as new mothers don't have to be flawless to be perfect. I recently had a conversation with a colleague whose children are now teenagers. As I shared my fears about returning to work and missing so much of my baby's life, I found myself in tears. She told me she had let perfection go a long time ago. She now sees herself as a B+ mom and a B+ professional because, as she put it, "You can't be an A in everything." Those words stung. I wanted to be an A+ mom for my baby. I needed to be. But in reflecting on her analogy, I realized there was something off about the grading system. What defines "perfect"? What truly deserves the highest grade? Let's explore this.

"Perfect" simply means to have all the required or desired elements. That's it. You have that within you, as does your baby. Do you have all that you desire at this moment? Maybe not, but what is "desired" is subjective. You can always seek more, but can you find peace in accepting what you have in this moment as enough?

What is your favorite moment from today? Hold on to that. Use it as a reminder of the mother you are becoming and let it lift you up when you need encouragement.

(A PRAYER FOR TODAY)

May I embrace, accept, and appreciate each moment for the gift that it is.

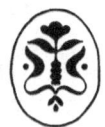

Sip of Self-Care:

Even when your hair is a mess on top of your head, you haven't showered in days, and you feel out of sorts, take a picture with your little babe. Capture the essence of this special time to look back on years from now. Your love story is just beginning, Mama. Let the sweet moments of your day be what you remember for years to come.

Forward is the only direction

Every story, every movie, every tale that captivates us has one thing in common: they're always moving forward. Even when the main character is struggling, those moments of challenge are essential to the storyline—and so it is with you. You are always moving forward, even when it feels hard.

You will feel different every single day, every single moment. Your body will go through phases. Your mindset will evolve, though some days, negative chatter will rear her ugly head. Your emotions might feel like an unpredictable roller-coaster ride, carrying you to heights and depths you didn't expect. And you know what? It's all okay because going back to who you once were is not the goal—and it's not going to happen. And honestly, would you even want to?

Instead, you will move *forward* into a whole new version of yourself in the exact place you are meant to be. You will experience strength, grace, and compassion like never before. Your confidence will take root as you continue to listen to your intuition and walk in soul alignment with who you are called to become.Forward is the direction of every meaningful story. And yours? It's unfolding beautifully, one chapter at a time.

(A PRAYER FOR TODAY)

When I feel the weight of change, grant me strength.

When my emotions rise and fall, bring me peace.

When negative thoughts cloud my mind, fill me with truth and clarity.

Help me to trust that every challenge, every moment of struggle, is part of the story you are writing with me.

Keep going, if only to see what happens

Your fears don't define you. In fact, I like to think of fear as courage in disguise, waiting to be recognized. Your missteps and mistakes don't break you. And they don't dictate the course of your life.

We've all felt fear or doubt, including every mother I know. However, something magical happens when we acknowledge our fears and our insecurities: we claim our power. We stand a little taller; we no longer outsource our inner knowing.

I know this time in your life can bring immense joy along with bouts of questions, what ifs, and moments of uncertainty. Every feeling you experience is valid. So, feel all of it. And then breathe it out.

One day, the mountain you are climbing will be behind you. But the person you've become in the climb—she will be within you forever. Perhaps, that's the true purpose of the mountain in the first place.

Keep going. You've welcomed this adventure into your life, and you're meant to embrace the fullness of its unfolding, wholeheartedly.

(A PRAYER FOR TODAY)

God, give me the wisdom to witness my fears, my anxieties, and my errors and to know that they do not define who I am. May I recognize each of them as a signpost guiding me toward what needs healing, embracing, or accepting.

Turn down the heat

I woke up this morning after a long night. I felt dysregulated and generally out of my body. I recognized that fire in my belly, and not the good kind that leaves you motivated; rather, it's the kind that results from being utterly exhausted. My mood could be described as "unpleasant," to say the least. And then, as I stepped into the shower, I felt it dissipate a bit. I got out, put on my favorite oil that has a hint of orange, and a little more steam released from my toes. I closed my eyes and took five long and deep inhales and exhales. And then I realized what I was doing with these small practices: I was turning down the heat.

It is perfectly normal to boil over because we, as mothers, are constantly keeping the fire alive in our house. But when it feels like too much, I invite you to pull back, even in small ways. Let go of the mess in the kitchen. Take a walk outside, light a candle, breathe.

In other words, use the things you *can* control to lighten the weight of the things you can't.

When your pot is boiling over, turn down the heat.

(A PRAYER FOR TODAY)

God, give me pockets of reassurance and peace that I am on the right pathway. When things are hard, remind me that I am also a vessel worth caring for and showering with compassion.

You matter

A nourished mother is the heart of a nourished baby and family.

This may sound like a cliché (like happy wife = happy life); however, there is truth to it.

You are the backbone, the landing pad, the safety blanket of your family. You are the thread that ties everything and everyone together. I know it might not seem like it sometimes, especially when you are caught up in the day-to-day just trying to make it through everything that comes your way. But a nourished you is a nourished baby and family. There is no other mother for your baby but you. It all starts with you.

Nourish yourself by not being the last one to eat your meal.

Nourish yourself by allowing help with the house, even if it's just once in a while.

Nourish yourself by taking time to rest with your baby, to soak up the moments.

In doing this, you "get on your own side" and build up your inner support system in the form of your health, your mood, and your energy.

You matter, Mama. Never forget how much.

(A PRAYER FOR TODAY)

In each moment, may I lean into nourishment. Of mind, body, soul. Of home and hearth.

Sip of Self-Care:

While the love and energy for your baby might be palpable, it's important to replenish yourself. A simple, nourishing ritual can be as easy as making a batch of sun tea. Here's a recipe to help you stay hydrated and feel grounded:

Sun Tea Recipe:

INGREDIENTS:

- 4–6 tea bags (your choice of herbal tea—chamomile, mint, or lemon balm are soothing options)
- 8 cups of filtered water
- A few fresh lemon slices (optional, for added brightness)
- A spoonful of honey or agave syrup (optional, for a touch of sweetness)

DIRECTIONS:

- Place the tea bags in a clean glass jar or pitcher.
- Pour the water over the tea bags and stir in the lemon slices, if using.
- Let the jar sit in a sunny spot for 3–4 hours, allowing the sun's warmth to gently infuse the tea.
- After steeping, remove the tea bags and add honey or agave syrup to taste, if desired.
- Pour over ice and sip throughout the day for a refreshing, hydrating boost.

As you sip your sun tea, take a moment to breathe, ground yourself, and nourish your soul.

You have permission to question it all

Don't be afraid to question it all. In your parenting, in your motherhood, in your relationships, in your passions. One thing I often remind myself is this: If you have a question, it deserves an answer. Too often we get inundated with propaganda, advertisements, and unsolicited advice from well-meaning friends, family members, strangers, and, of course, the media. And most of us tend to give in to the pressure of acquiescing and pleasing everyone around us.

But you're meant to see the world differently now with the new lens you've been given. And you don't have to stay in spaces and places that no longer feel aligned.

The why, what, and how are powerful questions to ask this season.

Why do I feel this way? *What* needs to change? *How* can I make this happen?

That last one (the *how*) always feels the most overwhelming for me. But the *how* is where we experience miracles. I love that reframe. The *how* is the way it unfolds *for us*. It's the surprising part of our story, of our journey.

So, ask all your questions without holding back. Don't be afraid to probe further, especially when it leads you to your dreams, to the aligned way of raising your family, to mothering your baby, and to advocating for your health and well-being. Follow that soul nudge, that nagging feeling that keeps you awake at night when you intuitively know *there is a better way to do this. There is something I am drawn to explore. There is a way that works for me and my family.* Be willing to venture out, away from the social norm. Be brave enough to find your own rhythm.

(A PRAYER FOR TODAY)

In moments of pressure, help me trust my inner knowing. It is safe to go against the grain and forge a path of my own—for me, my baby, and my family.

Finding peace in your choices

Celebrations, traditions, and holidays throughout the year can be whatever you make of them.

All the merry cannot be bright and cheery when you are anxious, overwhelmed, or already bracing yourself to navigate tricky family situations and dynamics.

I understand that adjusting to the rhythms of motherhood, especially with a new baby, can add another layer of challenge. But remember, these moments are yours to shape. Whether you host a large family gathering or just keep it intimate, the choice is yours. Don't hesitate to ask for what you need, whether that means skipping travel or keeping visits short. You are not obligated to meet anyone else's expectations at the cost of your peace of mind. Setting boundaries is not only okay, it's necessary for your well-being. These moments are yours to choose—whether you're embracing familiar traditions, creating new ones, or simply doing what feels best for you and your family. Let go of the pressure to conform to anyone's idea of how things "should be," and lean into the choices that bring you peace.

(A PRAYER FOR TODAY)

May this season be a time of peace, love, and kindness. Give me patience to witness people as they are and the wisdom and discernment to stay rooted in truth and love.

The compass of our body

A mother's body is a miraculous and intuitive force, always attuned to her baby's needs. For example, when breastfeeding, there are channels that allow saliva and backwash from the baby to reenter the mother's body, causing the alchemy of breastmilk to attune to exactly what the baby needs. Thus, if a baby is getting sick, the mother's body increases the number of leukocytes in her milk to boost the immunity of the baby.

Even if a mother is not breastfeeding, her body continues to experience hormonal changes that are connected to her baby's needs. The mere presence of her baby, the sound of their cries, or the act of holding them releases oxytocin, the "love hormone," deepening their emotional connection and reinforcing a mother's role as protector and guide.

Our bodies are deeply wise and truly amazing.

Your body subconsciously knows exactly what your baby needs. It's also a real-life thermostat for truth for honoring your voice, for honoring who you are and who you're becoming. Allow it to speak to you, to protect you, to warn you, to guide you.

Let your body guide you and your heart lead you.

Our vessel can act as our compass through every situation, if only we allow it to.

(A PRAYER FOR TODAY)

Thank you for my body and heart. Thank you for my innate intuition, my physiological responses that guide me on my journey.

Surrender wholeheartedly to the change ahead

I laid my baby on the bed today as I usually did, with his favorite giraffe teether in hand. It was a moment of respite while I folded laundry. Just a few seconds later, I heard a thud—slow motion and instant all at once. He'd rolled off the couch, his cry still echoing in my bones. I knew he was starting to roll, but not this soon, not with that much force.

Cortisol flooded my system. I felt like the worst mother in the world.

But after a breath and a calm moment, I shifted the narrative. I had been holding on to a version of my baby that he had already outgrown. It was a simple mistake, but a valuable lesson.

During this season in your motherhood, you're still freefalling into a whole new world. A whole new rhythm. What worked during these past few months of your baby's life may need tweaking as your baby learns new skills, passes new milestones, and grows in ways you may not be ready for (I know I'm not).

There are new routines, new systems, and new explorations taking place.

Surrender wholeheartedly to what is being asked of you. Give yourself the simple gift of not holding on so tightly.

You are almost six months wiser, more experienced and seasoned in this walk of motherhood.

Surrender into this season. Let it carry you, lifting you higher as you rise alongside your baby.

(A PRAYER FOR TODAY)

May I surrender into each day, each season, each act of devotion I am being asked to step into for myself, my baby, my body, my soul, my family.

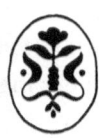

Sip of Self-Care:

A Ritual for Release

Light some candles, put on your favorite playlist (even if it's just for a song or two), and lie down on your bed. Beginning at the crown of your head, do a body scan, inviting each muscle in your body to release and soften. Let any worry cf heaviness drop off you. Notice how it feels to be completely held by the surface beneath you without needing to do anything at all.

A note on supporting mothers

Our current culture does not support mothers. I am realizing this more every day. As an eternal optimist, I never imagined how deeply this truth would hurt. Despite all the progress we've made, societal structures often neglect the unique challenges mothers face, and I will be the first to admit that until I became one myself, I couldn't really grasp all the pressure that falls on the shoulders of the mother trying to "do it all." From inadequate maternity leave policies to the lack of affordable childcare, the burden on mothers remains immense. The expectation that we balance full-time careers while being primary caregivers is unrealistic and unsustainable. But the more we speak out, the stronger our collective voice becomes.

Motherhood is not just a personal responsibility, it's a societal investment. Raising the next generation is essential work, work that should be recognized and supported. Yet mothers remain undervalued. To truly uplift families, we need extended paid leave, subsidized childcare, and flexible work policies. It's time for mothers to thrive, not just survive.

Here are a few ways to get involved and make change:

Advocacy: Raise awareness about maternal wellness and health policy needs through social media, community events, and supporting relevant organizations to influence public opinion and policymakers.

Policy Engagement: Contact and lobby local and national legislators to support maternity leave, childcare, and family-friendly policies through meetings, public comments, and coalitions.

Support Family-Friendly Businesses: Choose to work for or with companies that offer generous parental leave and family-friendly policies to set a standard and encourage others to follow suit.

Calm seas may bring peace, but it's in the storms we discover our power. And we are in the storm.

(A PRAYER FOR TODAY)

God, I pray for a society that embraces and supports mothers with the compassion and care they deserve. May we have the wisdom to create systems that value the essential role of mothers in nurturing the next generation. Help us build a world where we all feel uplifted, supported, and cherished.

The seven types of rest

Sleep is a commodity in motherhood. I think we can all agree that it's scarce and hard to find. But it gives me comfort knowing that sleeping is not the only way to rest. In fact, there are seven types of rest, and we need them all in varying degrees to feel truly rejuvenated. On days when I haven't gotten enough sleep, I look for other ways to incorporate the concept of rest into my day. Here are the different types and what they can look like for you:

Physical rest: lying down, mini naps

Mental rest: turning off your phone for stretches of the day or finding micro pockets of time to meditate

Emotional rest: spending time in your own energy field

Sensory rest: turning off the TV, putting down the technology, and walking outside in nature

Creative rest: playing with new hobbies, painting, or writing without expectation

Social rest: saying no when you need to and keeping a close circle in these early days

Spiritual rest: participating in daily prayer and readings that leave you feeling more connected to God

This list is by no means exhaustive so get creative today in other ways you can find pockets of rest. And I hope that this book provides some element of rest for you, Mama. Sending you so much love and ease today.

(A PRAYER FOR TODAY)

On days when it gets busy and the pressure feels heavy, help me remember that rest is my birthright and my deepest revolution as a woman, a mama, and a partner in a world that has forgotten what it means to feel truly rested.

Honor your ancestral lineage

Revere the women who came before you.

Your mother. Grandmother. Aunt. A wise woman. All have shaped your story in some way, and perhaps passed a piece of knowledge to you, either when you were growing up, in conversation, or in observation when you witnessed them lead/nurture/raise you and their own children. What wisdom have they imparted that you carry into motherhood?

As I reflect on my own journey, I am reminded of my mother's deep pride in her work as a first-grade teacher. To her, it wasn't merely a job—it was a calling, a purpose she embraced fully. She often told us that there was no greater gift than teaching someone to read. I still hear the voices of her former students, decades later, seeking her out to express their gratitude for the love and care she poured into them. Her example taught me the importance of passion in whatever path I choose and how love, woven into the fabric of our work, leaves an imprint that lasts beyond our lifetime.

She also taught me the healing power of forgiveness. No matter what mistakes we made, we knew that if we simply approached her with a hug, her heart would soften, anger would dissolve, and peace would always return. She couldn't hold a grudge if she tried. Her blend of passion and a forgiving spirit continues to guide my heart today.

Today, take a moment to send some loving energy and gratitude to the women who've gone before you. Even if those relationships are complicated to reflect on, know that their mere existence had some small part in leading you to where you are today, with your sweet baby in your arms. Hold them in your thoughts.

(A PRAYER FOR TODAY)

Thank you, God, for the wisdom of the women in my life, for my ancestors, and for the countless women who've gone before me.

Wander with an open heart and you will find your way home

Lean into your vulnerability. Fearlessly, without any guilt or shame. Vulnerability is your greatest strength. It's a heart opener—for you and your baby. Not every day will be perfect or without its fair share of overwhelm or anxiety-inducing moments. But it's in these moments that we owe it to ourselves and our soul to be honest, vulnerable, and transparent.

Leaning into your vulnerability can look like admitting you need support from friends or family, or even your partner. Letting someone into your heart takes courage and letting yourself be witnessed in your experience takes even more.

The root word of courage is "cor," which is Latin for "heart." And in Old French, the term "corage" meant "heart; innermost feelings," which reflects the idea that courage is an internal strength drawn from one's core self. Living with your whole heart, then, in this context, means embracing vulnerability and authenticity.

Your village is here to support you, but you have to let them in.

(A PRAYER FOR TODAY)

In moments when I resist opening my heart, may I always know and trust that my vulnerability is not a weakness but a strength.

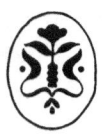

Sip of Self-Care:

Embrace the Truth of Your Journey

Give yourself permission to be fully honest about your feelings. Acknowledging both the highs and the lows of motherhood sends a powerful message to your inner self: there's nothing to hide, nothing to be ashamed of. Every emotion—joy, exhaustion, love, frustration—is a natural part of this transformative journey. By embracing your truth, you create space for healing, growth, and the deep knowing that you are enough, exactly as you are.

Cradle the cocoon

My son had a strong preference when it came to sleep; essentially, he only wanted to sleep when he was in our arms, preferably chest to chest. Lying next to my partner or me did not count in his eyes, as he wanted to be at an upright angle. It sounds specific, silly even as I reflect, but it was the truth of the moment. This meant that during the day, we were contact nappers. At night, my partner and I spent hours rocking, shushing, singing, and bouncing.

Often, as I was nestled in the embrace of exhaustion, I felt the invisible strands of sleep wrap around me like a spider's silk. My eyes would be heavy. In other moments, however, it seemed I was trapped by this growing web, my mind fluttering, yearning to break through and soar once more. If only I could get up, hands free, finish a few things I had on my mind, shower perhaps. The struggle to escape, to find a moment's respite, mirrored the futile dance of a fly ensnared by the intricate design of a patient weaver.

It's not easy to slow your pace to almost a halt for long periods of the day or night when you have been living at a high speed for most of your life. So, let me remind you today that it's okay to feel the whiplash from this new speed, anxious over the thought of being tethered once again to that special spot in your baby's room.

What helps me the most in these times is to close my eyes and picture myself as ninety years old. I'm likely sitting in a very similar chair. I imagine describing what this moment feels like to her. The weight of our baby on my chest, the thin layer of warmth between our bodies, the rhythmic sound of his breathing.

This, I remind myself, is metamorphosis, the heart of transformation. This is the cocoon. For it is here, in this quiet pause, that we are being remade.

(A PRAYER FOR TODAY)

God, teach me how to savor the moments in between. May I remember I am being planted into the most abundant season of my life.

To replicate or replace? That's the question.

How has your childhood influenced your motherhood?

We all pick up habits, behaviors, rituals, and traditions from our childhood. The experiences we've had growing up, the type of relationships we've witnessed within our families that raised us, they all play a role in shaping our worldview and influencing how we will parent our children. Positive and negative. There is no shame in this, only grace and compassion.

What are some positive parenting habits you've chosen to bring with you into this beautiful journey of motherhood? What are some habits or ways of parenting that you don't want to repeat, that end with you?

Take some time to sit with these questions. Ask the same of your close friends. It's always so interesting to see what comes up. Today, give thanks for all the golden glimmers you witnessed growing up; take those memories with you and forever cherish them and infuse them into your life with your baby and family. And for all the memories that might be heavy, honor their place in your story as they've shown you who you'd love to be as a mother and how you'd do things differently if given the chance. Now is your chance.

(A PRAYER FOR TODAY)

Give me grace and compassion when I reflect on my childhood. May I embrace each experience for what it was and what it taught me.

Focus on the small moments

What would you tell your baby about this moment in time? What has been your favorite memory so far in all these months? How would you describe it? You are a treasure trove of their memories, Mama—for you, for your baby, for your lineage and legacy.

As mothers, we all want to give our children the very best, but what does that mean? The consumer economy tells us we should be participating in playdates, scheduling social outings for our kids, going on grand adventures, and buying more things to provide our child with a happy childhood. But the truth is, they don't need all that.

Especially in these early years, our babies are just trying to figure out one thing: *Are they safe?* Safe to grow, explore, expand, and play? This is where their root chakra comes into play—the foundation of their sense of security and stability. The root chakra, located at the base of the spine, is the energy center that governs our feelings of safety, grounding, and connection to the earth. For your baby, the development of this chakra is vital to their emotional and physical well-being.

The core memories that build this foundation are made in moments of closeness—when you cuddle in the early hours of the morning, when they begin looking at you in a way that signals they really see and know you, and when you hear their first giggle. These moments may seem small, but they are powerful. They plant the seeds of trust and connection that will grow with your child as they navigate the world.

Remember this when it feels like you are stuck in the house or when you are juggling a job outside the home and mothering. When it all feels like a lot. Know that you are doing the very best you can. Focus on the small moments. They are the ones that truly matter. And in them, you are grounding your child's heart, nurturing their root chakra, and laying the foundation for a life full of love, security, and strength.

(A PRAYER FOR TODAY)

God, let me remember these moments not just for what they are, but for who we become as we live them.

The interplay between the third eye and your intuition

There are seven chakras or energy centers that run along the body. The sixth chakra, known as the third eye chakra, governs your intuition and is located right between your eyebrows. An open (or strong) third eye gives us the ability to observe the physical realm more clearly and provides "inner sight"—when we know something exists without it being visible.

This is your emotional intelligence. Your maternal instincts. What you feel in your heart. Trusting it and letting it lead you is everything because this is God's voice speaking to you in each moment—through your body, through those whispers.

You are the mother who was carefully selected for your baby. You are the only one who knows what is best for you both. Don't be afraid to trust your instincts and question a practice if you feel instinctively that it's not aligned with your mothering values. Share your voice and be the voice for your baby. You have been entrusted with this sacred responsibility.

Open and strengthen your third eye through supportive breathwork practices (see next page).

You are so powerful.

(A PRAYER FOR TODAY)

May I always know that it is safe to trust my intuition. It is safe to be a voice not just for myself but also for my baby.

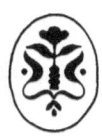

Sip of Self-Care:

Awaken Your Intuition with 4-7-8 Breathing

Tap into your inner wisdom by opening your third eye chakra with a grounding breathwork practice called 4-7-8 breathing. This technique activates your parasympathetic nervous system, shifting you into a calm, rest-and-digest state where intuitive insights can flow more freely.

1. Find a comfortable position where you can relax fully.

2. Begin by exhaling completely through your mouth, letting out all the air with a gentle "whoosh."

3. Close your mouth and inhale deeply through your nose for a count of four, imagining the breath filling your mind with clarity.

4. Hold your breath for a count of seven, letting the stillness settle your body and mind.

5. Exhale slowly and fully through your mouth for a count of eight, making an audible "whoosh" sound as you release tension and mental clutter.

Repeat this cycle ten times, moving at your own pace. With each breath, feel yourself becoming more aligned, centered, and open to the subtle intuitive messages within. Let this practice leave you feeling deeply settled and attuned to your inner knowing.

Love is the whole point

It all adds up, Mama. You are the great equalizer in this beautiful journey of motherhood.

In the endless nights when sleep eludes you, and in the moments when your human frailty shows—when you lose your cool or falter under the weight of it all—know that each experience is a thread in the rich tapestry of your journey. There are days when it feels like you're trapped in a never-ending cycle, and then there are others when your heart is so brimming with love for your baby that it feels like it might burst.

In those fleeting moments you wish you could pause and hold forever, and in the times when you beam with pride, feeling deep satisfaction despite the struggles, and the in-between, know that it is all part of your inner bloom. As you nurture your baby, you also nurture and transform yourself. You reparent yourself, giving the love you have longed for.

Can you see yourself, fully and lovingly, embracing every part of who you are?

Your firstborn is on this journey with you, growing and learning alongside you. They see you in your raw, unfiltered state, witnessing your tears and mistakes, and supporting you through the toughest times. They are a living testament to your growth and resilience.

Everything you do, every sacrifice, every moment of doubt and joy, all comes from a place of profound love. Love is your essence. You are balancing every challenge with the depth of your love.

(A PRAYER FOR TODAY)

Love is the equalizer in every moment. May I be love, see love, and lead with love.

You can be cracked open without being broken

God has a profound way of taking things that feel broken and filling in the cracks not just with healing but with something even more beautiful. Like the Japanese art of *kintsugi*, where broken pottery is carefully mended with gold. The fractures, instead of being hidden, are embraced as part of the object's history, creating something more exquisite and unique than before it was broken.

You, too, are a work of *kintsugi*. The cracks in your life, your heart, your journey—they are not signs of failure. They are evidence of resilience, love, and the healing touch of grace. With God's care, the very places that feel shattered can become the golden seams that tell a story of beauty, transformation, and strength.

I know that some days are challenging, and perhaps your experience of motherhood hasn't been typical. Most mothers I interviewed had some nuance they were facing that was individual to them and their family. Maybe you're navigating a critical-care or special-needs diagnosis, or perhaps you're in relationships that are falling apart. Or maybe you're experiencing postpartum depression or other physical challenges in your body as you continue to heal and bloom.

Know that you are not broken and your life is not broken.

Even if it feels like your world is crumbling. Know that even in those dim moments, God has a way of lighting up your life, your path. Healing isn't about erasing the cracks or pretending the pain isn't there. It's about honoring your story and allowing the fractures to be transformed into something useful. Like *kintsugi*, the golden seams of healing, love, and grace will run through your life, making you more radiant than you could have ever imagined.

Your story is far from over, Mama. Let it rearrange you.

(A PRAYER FOR TODAY)

Even in my lowest moments, I know you are with me. God, take the shattered fragments of my heart, of my life, of my challenges and pour your love onto them. Brighten my dark days with your peace.

Religion, politics, and . . . motherhood?

There is so much I love about motherhood, yet there is one thing I don't: how divisive it has become.

Are you breastfeeding or bottle feeding? Do you share your bed or use a crib? Home birth or hospital? Daycare or home with your baby? Nature school or public? Vaccinated or not?

These are the markers we use to judge whether we deem someone aligned with our own values. Subconsciously, we may even use them to decide whether *we* believe they are a "good mother." I don't claim to have all the answers, but here is what I know: Every woman I've met loves her baby fiercely, just like you do. And that love pulls us, beckoning us to rise to our tippy toes, to do the very best we can with what we have.

We were designed by God to be connected to our babies, first by body, but always by heart. Like osmosis, we hurt when they hurt, we feel what they feel, we laugh when they laugh.

I don't know a mother on this planet who thinks, *I really want to mess up today.* No.

She's reading, researching, talking to friends, comparing notes, racking her brain, lying awake contemplating options, and agonizing over decisions for her baby. She desperately wants to get it "right." She's gazing at her wide-eyed child, knowing that they are relying on *her.* Because that baby is hers. No one else's. No one loves her child the way she does. And for that reason, I do not care what choices you make for your own child. Because I know you are doing your best.

I know that because I see you, Mama. Don't let motherhood be another thing that divides us. Let it bring us together instead.

(A PRAYER FOR TODAY)

May my vision expand to embrace the beauty in every mother's journey. In my own path of nurturing, even when I falter, guide me to trust in my strength and wisdom, knowing I am exactly the mother my baby needs. Let each misstep become a stepping stone, each challenge a chance to learn.

Release all expectations

Expectations—we all have them. Of ourselves and others. We have expectations of how our loved ones should show up for us; of how we are supposed to show up as we continue to grow in our identity as a mother; of how our partnership or marriage is supposed to look and feel once we become parents; of how our friendships should feel on this new initiation. Expectations exist everywhere—overtly and covertly. And while they are great guidelines, that's all they are—guides.

The trouble unfolds when we unknowingly place our expectations on others and expect them to fulfill them instead of us embracing each other for who we are in each moment; instead of giving each other the grace of being human and leading with compassion for ourselves and each other. How much easier would that be? How freeing would that be? To know that you don't need to attend every single family celebration or constantly host gatherings, especially if you've been needing some quiet time with you, your baby, and your partner?

How freeing does it feel to know you have the power to choose which expectations you uphold and which ones you release and no longer subscribe to? Refreshing, isn't it! Release the expectation and see where you can be pleasantly surprised.

(A PRAYER FOR TODAY)

May I release the expectations that no longer serve me or any of my loved ones. I am free. I am enough.

Sip of Self-Care:

A Ritual of Release and Renewal

Today, step into the soothing warmth of a shower or bath, creating a sacred moment of care and connection. Begin by bringing your awareness to your body, starting at your toes. Offer each part of yourself a loving touch—whether a gentle squeeze, a tender stroke, or simply resting your hands with intention.

As you move slowly upward, through your legs, belly, chest, and arms, repeat softly: "The tension flows from my body, returning to the earth to be transformed into peace."

Feel the water washing over you, carrying away stress and fatigue. Imagine the earth beneath you receiving this release with grace, grounding you in its steady strength. As you reach your face, place your hands gently over your cheeks or heart and take a deep breath, welcoming the renewal this simple act has brought to your body and spirit.

Let this moment remind you that release is a gift you can offer yourself whenever you need it.

Your direction matters more than your speed

Before having my son, I was used to having a full calendar, and I honestly believed that once the initial shock and awe of motherhood faded, I would return to that speed. I couldn't have been more wrong. I was surprised by how much energy (and mental capacity for that matter) it required to even leave the house or venture somewhere new once I had a baby. My time was no longer my own. It was "our time," and it called for a different speed. Juggling multiple social events while scheduling appointments in the car between them was a thing of the past. With so much of my energy now focused on caring for my little one, I needed to simplify. And this wasn't just good for me, it was reassuring for him too.

Your baby is learning to explore more sounds and textures, familiarize themself with more voices, and relate to you and your partner, friends, grandparents, and/or other loved ones. This stimulation is incredible for their growth and development, *and* they need ample downtime to simply be. Space is the most beautiful gift you can give them, Mama. You will know when they're overstimulated. You will know when they instinctively don't want to be held or touched by anyone else.

Let their body cues, and your intuition, guide you. Let them bask in the unfolding of each day—freely, without constraint, in full safety that they are loved and their personal space is respected.

(A PRAYER FOR TODAY)

Teach me how to honor the moments in between when pleasing people doesn't run my world. Guide me on my path as I continue to learn and lean into new standards for myself and my family

Just because you can't see it, doesn't mean it's not there

I walked out into the brisk, sunlit morning and let out a sigh, baby on my hip. It was freezing, so my breath was visible in the cold air. I could tell my baby was interested. I stopped and I smiled. What a miracle to see our own breath. Too often I forget it's there.

And then it had me thinking about all the breaths we take that we don't see— all 22,000 of them that we have every day, humming in the background. We are so focused on everything we need to accomplish on our to-do list—the mother load, as I like to call it—that we sometimes forget to really expand our lungs and breathe.

So right now, let's remember together.

Inhale peace, exhale tightness.

Inhale love, exhale all that you're holding on to.

Inhale joy, exhale dimming out who you are.

Inhale calm, exhale anxiety. Release everything you're not in control of. It doesn't deserve space in your mind. Focus on the breath. Focus on how it feels in your body. Come back to this practice daily.

I like to take at least two minutes every day to remind myself to focus on my breath. Breathing is our most natural state of being, yet we forget to access it with awareness whenever life gets busy.

So deep, slow breaths daily, Mama.

(A PRAYER FOR TODAY)

God, thank you for every breath I take. Thank you for my heart that beats with so much life and love.

Look how far you've come

Not so long ago, your baby was just a single cell, a tiny spark of life. Can you believe that your body took two half cells and, over 280 days, transformed them into 26 billion cells? That's the incredible journey that brought you the baby you hold in your arms today.

Now here you stand, having cared for another being earthside with your full heart and soul for six months in which your baby has grown in every way—their body, their mind, their personality.

You've made it through the first six months, the ones often considered the hardest (although, let's be real, every part of motherhood is an adventure).

As you step into the next chapter, get ready for more beautiful firsts: their first crawl, their first steps, their first birthday, their first words, and so many more.

Celebrate yourself, your baby, and all that you've made it through. You're doing it, Mama.

(A PRAYER FOR TODAY)

Thank you, God, for these beautiful first six months with my baby. I embrace the next six months with a curious and open heart. I am always arriving, forever becoming.

God is working in your waiting

Most days I feel like I am on one of those moving walkways at the airport. There is a quiet movement under my feet, escorting me from one task to the next. However, in those moments when the house is still, and I have hopped off the conveyor belt for a few moments, I can feel how much I have changed. I sense that I am in this in-between phase, the gray space, where I am no longer the woman I was before birth but am also still finding my footing in motherhood. Will I one day just fully stand up? Or is this process a lifelong journey of stumbling and finding ourselves once again? I don't know. But I am trying to enjoy the space in between where I was and where I am going.

In these moments, God is showing us something because there is so much to learn as we wait for the next season to unfold. The pressure, the joy, the uncertainty, the love—they are all preparing us for what lies ahead. God is truly at work in our waiting.

(A PRAYER FOR TODAY)

God, in the midst of our waiting, we find comfort in knowing that your loving hand is at work. It's during these times of uncertainty and anticipation that we can see glimpses of your plan unfolding. We trust in your perfect timing, and with each passing day, we discover the beauty of patience, learning to lean on you and find strength in the assurance that you are working everything together for our good. Thank you for the lessons and growth that come with the waiting, and for the hope that it brings.

Sip of Self-Care:

Steeping in Stillness: A Tea Ritual for Reflection

Tea is more than a warm drink—it's a plant ally, offering its grounding energy and ancient wisdom to support you. Choose your favorite tea, one that feels like it can hold space for you in this moment. As the tea steeps, notice its aroma, its warmth, and the way the leaves transform the water.

Set a timer for five minutes and sit quietly with your tea. Breathe deeply, tuning into your five senses. Feel the warmth of the cup, the taste of the tea, the way it anchors you to the present. Imagine the tea as a companion, working gently with God to nourish your heart, mind, and soul. Let this moment remind you that rest is sacred and growth often begins in stillness.

When you're ready, reflect on your journey with these three questions:

- What are you most proud of so far?
- What has been one of your biggest lessons?
- Where do you feel called to lean into your growth edge in this season of motherhood?

Let the tea remind you that, like the plants it comes from, you are deeply rooted yet always growing—nourished by stillness, reflection, and divine love.

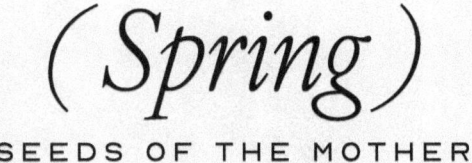

(Spring)

SEEDS OF THE MOTHER

THE THIRD QUARTER:

GROWTH, EXPERIMENTATION, RENOVATION

"The maiden is cultivated by what surrounds her,
the mother cultivates her surroundings."

Scan for meditations to guide you
through this season

Spring: Seeds of the Mother

GROWTH . EXPERIMENTATION . RENOVATION

In the Spring season, we are planting and watering the seeds of our reborn lives as mothers. To do this, we need the awareness and clarity to choose *which* seeds to plant and the energy to tend to those we have decided to sow. What then is the recipe, you may ask, to cultivate clarity and energy? Here are the three main ingredients:

Contemplative Practices: During contemplation practices like meditation and prayer, we can sift through the noise and unburden the mind long enough for the blurry edges of the past six months to truly come into focus. This season is an invitation to create a nurturing environment for the things we want to expand. Contemplative practices don't have to be long, but giving yourself some space, even micro moments of connecting to the breath, will go a long way to tap into what is meant *for you* in this period.

Movement: When we are undergoing a season of change and new beginnings, we tend to *feel* a lot, and if we aren't intentionally moving them up and out when we have a wide range of emotions, they can become stuck inside the body. Our emotions are simply "energy in motion"—they are meant to flow through us. Whether it means going for a long walk or just committing to an evening stretch, we need to move each day in some way.

Nature: God is in nature and nature *is* God's work in a physical, tangible form. When we step outside to absorb the beauty and miracle of life that is all around us, we further infuse God into our lives, our choices, and our life framework. When we are connected to God, we understand that we are never alone; this gives us strength to endure hard moments because our faith (in the form of waiting) resides on the other side of that pain. Let nature be a reminder during this season of the intricacy and beauty that is woven into all beings, including you.

Let this season be one of experimentation. Try things on and test things out but continue to anchor back to your budding motherly intuition and listen to your heart space to see what is right for you *now*. In the Mother Year, we are particularly raw, vulnerable, and in some ways, susceptible. While we cannot always control the outcome in a given situation, we can control the inputs into our mind, body, and soul. The seeds of your life will come in all shapes and sizes. Celebrate the small wins as those can often escalate into outsized imprints in your life.

It was during this season that I connected with a new friend. We had met briefly on a surface level on a prior occasion, but when she reached out to connect deeper, I felt a very clear ping of "yes." Truthfully, before meeting her, I had a strange idea that my deepest friendships had already been made (silly, I know). I had a great group of friends from different chapters in my life and genuinely felt like my cup was pretty full in that department. I was wrong. Within a few conversations with this woman, I felt so incredibly seen and held, and to this day, I consider her one of my closest friends. Our friendship was a seed and we watered it often. It started small but has now become one of the brightest and most flourishing relationships I have. A few texts quickly turned into long walks, phone chats after the babies went to bed, and uplifting messages. She is honest and kind and helps reflect the strength and beauty in my journey back to me.

Motherhood is an experience without a set mold or defined path. There is no universal guide, and that's what makes it so deeply personal. Each woman is different, as is each child, so your mothering will inevitably look different as well. And that is okay. This individuality is something to embrace, as it brings richness and authenticity to your story. The Spring season is time to reimagine your life and the parts that make it up. One journal entry from this period still lingers in my mind: *Find the balance of giving of yourself and keeping yourself.* In motherhood, it's easy to let the needs, wants, and dreams of others take center stage. It's also easy to set aside our own aspirations, using motherhood as a reason to wait. Only you know what you need to find joy and purpose in during this time, and whatever decision you make will be the "right" one as long as you walk forward in conscious choice.

You are evolving and growing, even in the moments that don't feel as if you are, even on those days when you feel low vibrations and are just trying to make it through. Like a caterpillar, slowly and steadily shedding its cocoon, your metamorphosis is underway. These new beginnings create new opportunities to create a life where you flourish as the incredible mother you are.

I hope this Spring season brings you:

- Colors that touch your heart
- Creative ideas that surprise you
- Clarity to quit what is not working
- Courage to move on from the past
- Confidence to go with your gut (your sacral center and authority)

You've got this, Mama.

Find your pockets of protected time

The 6 a.m. hour or the silent midnight reverie? That is the real question these days, isn't it? How do we find the time for ourselves, that precious time?

For me, it still feels hard to find areas of protected time, even though I know I need them now more than ever. I end up staying up late to write in my journal, record a voice note about the day, or watch an episode of my favorite show, then inevitably feel some level of guilt when I wake up tired the next day. Alternatively, I sometimes get up early to get my day started before my son wakes up but then am so tired by midafternoon that I begin questioning whether it was worth it. I am still finding my rhythm but know it is helpful to remind myself often that these clusters of time are never a "waste" (my patriarchal conditioning says that I must be productive).

Sunrise mornings for me are best spent meditating, reading a short reflection, praying, and in devotion time with God. And sometimes, when my stream of creativity does occur, it floods through in late-night reveries. This balance is what brings me peace on days when I feel restless; my pace is unhurried, almost as if I am standing in place. These pockets of time when I can ground and re-center remind me of my passions, my desires, and my interests; and in all honesty, they remind me that I am still a woman outside of motherhood.

Wherever you find yourself during this season of late nights or early mornings, choose the one that works for you. Find your pockets and walk with petals spilling out from your soul, Mama. You are worthy of it.

(A PRAYER FOR TODAY)

Wherever I find myself, early mornings or sleepless nights, teach me to find you in the silence, dear God. Pour creative, quiet reflection through me.

Your presence is potent

Your presence is what matters most, Mama.

Years from now, when your baby is all grown up, they will not remember if your house looked like a magazine spread or a cozy, lived-in space. What they'll hold on to is the love that surrounded them, the marks on the wall that celebrated their growth, and the joyful chaos that made their childhood feel *alive*.

It doesn't matter if your hair is messy or if yoga pants and sweatshirts have become your uniform. What your child will remember is your warmth, your snuggles, the way your voice soothed their fears, and your full-bellied laughter when they made you smile. On the tough days, when it feels like you're not doing enough, remind yourself that you are. Like a sunflower instinctively turning toward the sun, you are hardwired to turn toward your baby. That connection is everything.

So, give yourself permission to simply *be*—to embrace the mess, the moments, and the magic of the here and now. Because your love, Mama, is the greatest gift of all.

(A PRAYER FOR TODAY)

May my presence always be felt—in all that I am, all that I do, and everywhere I go.

Embracing the many versions of you

Right now, in this moment, who are you called to be as a mother, a partner, a woman?

Some days, the career-driven, mission-oriented woman appears in moments of peace and quiet. On other days, I'm lucky if I feel motivated to get out of bed. Some days, I miss going downtown to an office. On others, I dream of living on open land with chickens and a few goats. Some days, I crave adult conversations. Others, I just want to cuddle up and snuggle with my baby.

Wherever you find yourself, know that who you are in this moment is exactly who you need to be.

Honor the versions of yourself that surface throughout each day. In this season of motherhood, it is normal to feel pulled in different directions and for your mind to be trying out new versions of what life could look like for you. It's normal for your inspiration to wax and wane. Allow the inconsistency of how you feel day-to-day, week-to-week to be okay.

You are multidimensional, with a heart full of love and a mind full of God's visions planted in you—for you and your baby. In each moment when you feel guilt, "not enoughness," lack, worry, or anxiety pop up, ask yourself: Which aspect of me do I need to honor today?

Sit with her. Pray over her.

(A PRAYER FOR TODAY)

May I revere each version of me that wants to be seen, heard, and witnessed. In every passing moment.

Spring is in the air

Who doesn't love the arrival of spring? The buds breaking through the soil remind us of nature's incredible resilience and boundless potential, and this season of renewal can mirror your own journey through motherhood. Your little one is discovering their toes and giggling in pure delight, embodying the essence of the happy baby pose. For me, these moments marked the first inklings of ease in my motherhood journey. It was then I realized that the long, cold winter wouldn't last forever. I began to see signs of renewed life within myself, feeling the first stirrings of joy and possibility.

With my baby in tow, I started venturing out of the house and back into the world, feeling more connected and confident. I began to envision my potential as a mother, seeing glimpses of the strength and love I could bring to my child's life. Perhaps you are beginning to see signs of your own possibilities too.

How can you protect and nourish these tender sprouts of hope, ensuring they flourish and grow? Take a moment to appreciate the small victories and remember that you are doing more than you realize. You are cultivating a garden of love and care, not just for your little one, but for yourself as well. So today, let me remind you that your efforts are seen, your love is felt, and you are doing an incredible job. Keep nurturing those budding hopes and dreams, for they are the foundation of a beautiful future.

(A PRAYER FOR TODAY)

God, allow me to see and celebrate the signs of my growth as a mother.

Sip of Self-Care:

Notice the Beauty around You

Step outside or into a nearby garden, park, or even your own yard, and pick a flower, leaf, or sprig of greenery that catches your eye. Take a quiet moment to really look at it—notice the intricate textures of the petals, the vibrant or subtle colors, and the delicate veins running through the leaves or stems.

Let this natural beauty serve as a reminder of what's quietly blooming within you today. Like the flower, your growth may feel subtle, but it's full of detail and wonder. Carry this thought with you as you move through your day—small moments of beauty can reflect the transformation happening within.

Shed what is no longer in alignment with you or your baby

It's okay to shed the behaviors, people, situations, jobs and careers, and friendships and relationships you have outgrown.

I know the guilt creeps in from time to time . . .

But I've known ____ for years . . .

But I've worked here for so long . . .

But they're family . . .

But we've been best friends since grade school . . .

But this is how it's always been . . .

But this is ME . . . who I've always been . . .

The guilt is most likely laced with a tinge of fear, fear of who you are without the identity you've worn and held on to your whole life, be it in relationships, behaviorally, socially, or professionally. Give yourself permission to release, to evolve, to step into the momentum of the Mother Year and the transformations it's ushering in. Who you were before motherhood brought you here, but that past self may not have all you need for the path ahead. This is uncharted territory, Mama, and only you, your body, and your intuition can be the compass. The defenses and behaviors that once protected you may not serve you now, especially when you're focused on nurturing a legacy of love, not passing down pain.

Letting go of what no longer aligns is a profound act of self-love, one that nourishes your soul and sets the foundation for future generations to thrive. Embrace the shedding—it's the essence of your growth and the beginning of a whole new map.

(A PRAYER FOR TODAY)

Thank you for the wisdom of my mind, body, and soul—it helps me discern and shed what no longer is in resonance with who I am called to be. May I release with grace and compassion. Thank you for every person, every opportunity, and every experience that has made me who I am now. It is safe to make room for newness. It is safe to take up space and release everything I've outgrown.

Your choices around work don't make you less of a mother

Perhaps you have returned to work and you feel anxious, worried, and overwhelmed. Perhaps you are contemplating a power pause in your career. Perhaps you are exploring a new job or starting a business. Perhaps you can stay at home full-time with your baby.

Wherever you find yourself, it is completely normal to experience turbulence as you settle on what feels right for you. There are already so many changes swirling around us in new motherhood that choices around work can sometimes feel like an added layer of stress. I didn't anticipate how much I would love being home with my baby, so I was hesitant about returning to work. And once I did return and was able to get back into a flow, I wondered what it said about me that I *could* be without my baby for hours every day. Deep, contemplative feelings appeared at every turn. Reminding myself of these simple truths got me through this period:

Back to work doesn't mean you don't love your baby. And being home with your baby doesn't mean you're not driven, ambitious, or have a desire to provide for your family. Be gentle with yourself as you navigate changes in your capacity.

Wherever you are, know you are loved for who you are—not what you do. And these choices are nuanced in a way that no one else but you can truly appreciate.

(A PRAYER FOR TODAY)

Teach me how to release the guilt that surfaces as I weave in a new routine, a new cadence, a new part of my life into motherhood.

Starting solids

If you asked me what was filling up my headspace today, the answer would roll off my tongue with ease: food. But not for me—for my baby.

During this season, many of us are faced with what feels like monumental choices around introducing food to our little ones. Should I start with baby-led weaning or purees? What should I feed them first? Does my baby have an allergy? How do I prevent my baby from choking? Is this too big a piece of food? Or is this too small? How much should they be eating, and how often? Are they getting enough nutrients?

These questions swirl around constantly, making every mealtime feel like a high-stakes exam. And it's exhausting. I truly get it.

It *will* get easier with time, so don't rush it. Trust your instincts and embrace the messy, imperfect moments. Every "meal" is a step forward—a new experience for your baby, and a new lesson for you. It's okay if your baby makes a mess or if they reject certain foods. It's all part of the process. You're learning together and there is something beautifully profound in that. I even started a list on my phone of foods my baby had tried, a little reminder of the adventure unfolding in their world. I'm aiming for one hundred foods by the end of the first year—just for the fun of it and to celebrate all the tiny milestones along the way.

Remember, every baby is different. What works for one might not work for another, and that's perfectly normal. It's not about following a strict set of rules but rather about finding what works best for you and your little one. Some days will be easier, and others might be more challenging, but that's the ebb and flow of motherhood.

Celebrate the small victories, like the first time your baby tries a new food or the joyful messes they create. These moments, as chaotic as they may seem, are fleeting and precious. Enjoy the journey, one bite at a time.

(A PRAYER FOR TODAY)

Thank you for allowing me to savor the steps in feeding my precious baby. I feel very grateful to be able to provide for them.

A mother like no other

There is beauty in every imperfection, every mess, every scar. In every harrowing experience that rocks you and brings you to your knees. In those evening hours when you are being stretched. In the never-ending days and the sleepless nights. In the evolution of your relationship with your partner. In the oodles of pump parts, baby bottles, and burp rags that have taken over the decor of your house. There is beauty everywhere, if you allow yourself to witness it and experience it.

The clearest reflection of this beauty is the little being in front of you. When you look at your baby, no matter how much they may keep you up at night or spit-up on you, no matter how much they cry when they are having a hard moment, you accept them completely, love them fully.

Can you offer yourself grace in the same way?

A reminder today that you don't have to be a flawless mother, you just have to be a loving and present one, which you already are. You are growing in these moments, little by little, breath by breath.

Just like in early spring, when the seed is just awakening, you are in a season of change, of revival. It may not be obvious to the outside world, but it's happening underneath the surface of your skin, within your mind, a new muscle memory for your heart.

Today, embrace the imperfections. A rose does not long to be any other flower but itself. It blooms in its own time, in its own way. Let your life be one of your own variety. A bloom like no other. A mother like no other.

(A PRAYER FOR TODAY)

Teach me to see the beauty in all things great and small. In the grit and the glory.

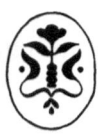

Sip of Self-Care:

Celebrate Small Wins: A Bedside Reflection

At the end of each day, take a moment to reflect. Write down or record a voice note capturing one small victory or lesson from the day. It doesn't need to be monumental—maybe you stayed patient in a stressful moment, paused to take a deep breath, or carved out a sliver of time just for yourself.

These small wins are the stepping stones of your growth. By honoring them, you're not just acknowledging your journey—you're lifting it up, piece by piece. Over time, these moments will weave together, showing you just how far you've come. Let this nightly practice be a quiet celebration of the progress unfolding within you.

The power of pouring into yourself

You cannot pour from an empty cup.

The people I know who care for themselves are stronger, kinder, and wiser because their inner capacity has increased. In some ways, this feels counterintuitive to me—the idea that taking time to pour into myself allows me to pour more abundantly on my baby. But it's true. You have to "have" in order to give.

Filling up your chalice, your own cup, doesn't make you selfish. It makes you self-aware. It means you're attuned to the whispers of your mind, body, and soul. It allows you to be fully YOU, the mother your child needs most.

In what ways can you pour back into yourself this season so that your light can burn brighter?

(A PRAYER FOR TODAY)

God, fill up my cup in ways only you can do.

Heart talk is the most genuine conversation that exists

Did you know that when you and your baby gaze into each other's eyes, exchanging smiles, your heart rhythms harmonize, syncing within mere milliseconds of each other. This phenomenon, known as "biological synchrony," reflects a profound communication style unique to mothers and babies.

Your heartbeat is so powerful—it's more than a rhythm, it's a force of life.

Be it your sacred yes or a sacred no, honor it with your heart.

Love fiercely with every beat of your heart.

Forgive freely with a heart wide open.

Seek to understand yourself and others within the depths of your heart.

Forge your path as a mother with all your heart.

God gave you this initiation, this beautiful baby. This sacred responsibility and divine assignment.

Step fully into who you are meant to be according to the wisdom of your heart. Let it be the compass that guides you. All the way.

(A PRAYER FOR TODAY)

Lead me, guide me, move with me—in my heart, in my words, in my visions, in my actions.

Walking with duality

Every day brings a blend of experiences that rarely fit neatly into categories. Some days we feel the pull of duality more intensely, living in the tension of opposing truths.

But motherhood, like life itself, is rarely black or white. Sometimes we battle challenges in our motherhood that nobody knows a thing about—strained relationships, workplace conflicts, or the weight of family illnesses or drama.

Whatever it is you are walking through, know that it will not last forever. Within this complexity lies a profound truth—the gift of nuance.

Peace may coexist within moments of sadness or chaos. Hardship often reveals glimmers of ease. Abundance and overflow make space for clearing and release.

Motherhood is the dance of duality—the interplay of light and shadow, the ebb and flow of challenge and grace. It is the practice of revering what each contrast teaches us, finding strength in both the grit and the gentleness.

You are capable, you are enough, and while it may feel like you're exploring the vastness on your own, know that God walks with you, beside you. Your village stands ready with open arms, waiting to support you as you find your stride in this nuanced, sacred path.

(A PRAYER FOR TODAY)

God, give me the courage to dance with duality, to honor it, to face it with grace and strength.

It works if it works for you and your baby

Crip or co-sleep? Breastfeed or formula? What is the right route to take?

The real answer is, whatever is best for you and your baby.

Every culture is different, every family is nuanced, and every baby has unique aspects about them.

For example, my son didn't sleep well in bed with us but also didn't want to be in another room without us. In his perfect world, he would be chest to chest while being rocked all night, something we did for months until I could barely see straight. I read all the books, talked to sleep consultants, and drove myself crazy trying to "crack the code." In the end, we developed a special routine that combined nursing, rocking, rubbing his chest in this crib, holding his hand, singing to him, and a host of other concoctions. An alchemy of sleep support that worked *for him.* The details of our sleep journey really don't matter, though. This decision is more than just one about sleep, it's about listening to your own inner compass.

Wherever you find yourself, know that you should do works for you and your family. That's all that matters. And only you will know when something needs to change or when you are ready to invite in advice from others. I hope you feel empowered today to make the choices that work for *you.*

(A PRAYER FOR TODAY)

God, help me lean into the most supportive decisions for my baby and me as we both deepen our walk together.

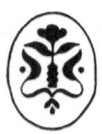

Sip of Self-Care:

Next time you're in a state of decision paralysis (today or in the days to come), repeat:

"I make decisions with the best information I have. I'm learning, and together, my baby and I will find the right path forward, even if there are twists and turns along the way."

The melody of your motherhood

Discover your soul beat—live, breathe, and mother to a rhythm as multidimensional as you.

Music has a way of moving us, reaching into the deepest parts of our being. Science tells us that music activates more areas of the brain than almost any other activity, stirring emotion, sparking memory, and even deepening our connection to others. This has always been clear to me when I turn on a song of worship or healing frequencies. Without fail I am moved to tears as I sing along; it's as if spirit is woven into the melody, calling us home. Your soul song is no different; it's yours, sacred, unique, and alive.

You don't need to be like anyone else or follow someone else's rhythm. Those are just ideas born from what worked for them. You're in the process of identifying and refining what works best for you and your baby. Sometimes the pitch and key will change; other times, it will be a familiar tune. But it will always be your song.

Lean into it and let it guide you. And know that it's okay if this period of growth feels immense—neither you nor your baby has ever danced to this rhythm before.

You're composing the melody as you go, each note a testament to your unfolding story. You're getting to know a new side of yourself, one that is both softer and stronger. Feel the textures, the context, and the layers of this current season. This is your time to discover the parts of yourself that lie beneath the surface—the foundation of your being—longing to be reawakened on this journey.

(A PRAYER FOR TODAY)

Let me sing the song of my soul, daily. Whether the pitch is off-key or catchy or a soothing lullaby, it is a song in my heart, my actions, my love for my baby.

Embody being present

I love how Corrie ten Boom so beautifully compares prayer to the soul as wings to a bird.[11]

Imagine yourself standing at the edge of a vast, quiet lake at dawn, birds flying above. The surface is so still it mirrors the sky. You take a step closer, and the moment your toes touch the water, it ripples. Not in chaos, but in response, as if it recognizes your presence.

This is embodiment.

It's being so present in your body, your heart, and your soul that even the world around you seems to respond.

What really matters to you most right now? Focus on that. Let yourself be there, wholly.

It's easy to get swept up in other people's agendas about how you should mother, spend your time, care for your baby, and nourish your own body, mind, and soul. But embodiment means stepping out of the noise and back into the truth of your own skin, your own breath. It means rooting yourself so deeply in the moment that you can hear the voice of your soul—God's voice—guiding you. Let this be your moving prayer of embodiment.

Every time you pause to feel the ground beneath you, to listen to what is truly calling you, you are living this prayer. In that stillness and response, you hold the power of presence, the power to mother from a place of your own divine connection.

Let it remind you that you are whole, rooted, and exactly where you need to be.

(A PRAYER FOR TODAY)

God, guide my heart and presence to what matters most in this moment. To what my baby and I most need.

A word on innate intelligence

Just because you have help and support does not mean you don't *know* your baby. Don't undermine your innate knowing as their mother.

When I went back to work and had to explain in detail to our nanny how to care for my baby, I realized something extraordinary: I could practically write a manual on my child. Every cry, coo, and expression—what they wanted, what they needed, how they felt—it all lived in me, like a map etched into my heart. That's when I understood that the intelligence I had developed as their mother was nothing short of genius.

But here's the thing: this innate intelligence isn't just ours as mothers. Our babies come into this world equipped with their own kind of brilliance. They know how to communicate before they can speak, how to find comfort in our arms, how to teach us about themselves through subtle cues. They are our partners in this journey, born with the wisdom to guide us just as we guide them.

Have you ever doubted just how deeply you know your baby? Or perhaps those more experienced around you (unknowingly, unintentionally) made you doubt your innate intelligence?

It can be easy to second-guess yourself, but remember that your body created and birthed this being. You know them in ways no one else ever will.

You were built especially for them, and they you. Your connection isn't just instinct, it's a shared knowing that is as ancient as motherhood itself. Trust it. Trust *yourself.*

(A PRAYER FOR TODAY)

God, may I cultivate a deeper sense of self-trust as I journey deeper into motherhood.

You are enough

I'll never forget the first time my baby truly noticed me. He was just a few months old, lying on his play mat, kicking his tiny legs in delight. I leaned over, smiling down at him, and in an instant, his whole face lit up with a grin so radiant it felt like it could outshine the sun. In that moment, I realized something profound. I wasn't just his mother, I was his whole world.

Motherhood has a way of making us question ourselves, doesn't it? I can't count how many times I felt like an impostor, typing frantic questions into Google at 2 a.m., convinced I was doing it all wrong. But here's the truth I wish I could go back and whisper to that version of me: "Those little eyes see so much more than you think."

Your baby isn't measuring your mistakes or keeping score. They are soaking in every single word you speak, every tune you hum, every hug and every snuggle—every memory you co-create with them.

You are their mother, their protector and best friend; their very first everything. It's through you and from you they learn to connect, relate, and love themselves and the world around them.

So, on the days when you're wondering if you're really cut out for this, when the weight of motherhood feels heavy on your shoulders, let this be your reminder: You are exactly what your baby needs. You are their safe haven, their comfort, their hero.

And that radiant grin? It's their way of saying "You're doing just fine, Mama. I chose you."

You are more than enough.

(A PRAYER FOR TODAY)

Thank you for this gift of being my baby's hero. There will be days when I make mistakes, days when I have absolutely no clue how we will make it through. Still, my baby loves me and trusts me. May their innate love and trust in me help me trust myself more. May I see myself through the eyes and heart of my baby.

Sip of Self-Care:

Take a moment to rub your hands together, feeling the warmth you create with this simple act. Then, gently place your hands on your baby, letting that warmth flow into them. This is a reminder of the power you carry—your energy, your love, your presence. No one else can provide this unique connection. You are their protector and whole world. Let this touch be a reminder that your love is more than enough.

Sowing the life you deserve

Society has long sold us the myth that our worth lies in constant hustle, that joy is something to be fought for, and that rest is a luxury—or worse, a weakness. The old adage, "You can sleep when you're dead," couldn't be further from the truth.

But here's what I want you to know: You *can* have the life your soul craves. Motherhood. Deep, nourishing relationships. Creative outlets that light you up. Expansion in every way that feels aligned for you and your family. It's all possible—but first, you have to let go. Let go of the rigid timelines, of how it's supposed to unfold, and the "shoulds" society places on you. You need to march to the beat of your own heart.

After having my son, I made a bold move. I switched jobs to work remotely, a decision rooted in my longing for more time at home. But soon, I found myself missing connection and craving community, so I started leading Mothers' Circle gatherings once a month. They began small, intimate, almost hesitant. But they grew and so did I. Some of those women are now my closest friends.

It wasn't instant, know that. It was more like an unthawing, a gradual awakening of the parts of me that had been quietly dormant since becoming a mother. I started watering those pieces. Not all at once, but slowly over time. And they looked much different than they had before I became a mother. Each time I felt that ping of comparison, I looked to see what it was about that lifestyle I found desirable. Bit by bit, I planted those seeds of my own.

It's a work in progress. I'm still planting, still tending, and I hope you are too. Because this is how we grow the lives we dream of—not by sprinting, but by sowing. Seed by seed, day by day.

(A PRAYER FOR TODAY)

God, I surrender my timeline to you. Let everything unfold in your time, not mine. I trust the woman and mother I am becoming every single day.

Your baby knows you love them

Trust me, they do.

Even when you're overwhelmed,
Or step away to catch your breath.
Even when the weight of it all feels heavy,
And sadness sits quietly beside you.

Even when you're wondering how you'll keep going,
Grieving the you that's now a memory.

Even when joy bubbles over,
As they snuggle close and reach for the world.

Even when you're their source of life,
Feeling more like a milk factory than a muse.

Even when you carve out space for yourself,
To remember who you are beyond them.

Even when you chase the calling of your heart,
Balancing love and purpose with every step.

Your baby knows you love them.
Not because of perfection,
But because love lingers in the spaces between—the waning chaos, the
radiant mess.
The everything you are and all you give,
Even when you doubt it.

Your baby knows you love them.
Your love hums in their very bones,
A melody they'll carry long after these moments are a memory.

(A PRAYER FOR TODAY)

*May I remember that my baby knows I love them. My love is enough. It is everything.
May I hold this truth in my heart always, in each moment, near and far.*

You are the bridge between worlds

My favorite question in the meditation teacher trainings I lead is: How are you a bridge?

The answers people give are fascinating. We are all a bridge in some way or another, in our families, our work, our friendships.

Right now, you are certainly a bridge for your baby as you walk between two worlds—yours and theirs.

That is the power that you wield in your field, Mama.

You are the harbinger of life, the one who sustains, nourishes, nurtures, and thrives, no matter the conditions or circumstances.

You are their link to God and the one who helps them walk tall and rooted in their soul, here on earth.

As you continue to step into your emboldened motherhood, remember this: You are the golden thread between two worlds—yours and theirs. Heaven and Earth. Soul and Body. Conscious and Unconscious.

You are powerful beyond measure, and this thing we call motherhood is quite possibly the greatest adventure of all.

(A PRAYER FOR TODAY)

God, plant my feet firmly in the knowing that my motherhood has a greater purpose. That I am the golden light that connects them to me, to you, and to the rest of the world.

Home is wherever I am with you

For your baby, home is wherever they are *with* you.

I'll never forget a night when my son was just a few months old. We were traveling, and he had a hard time settling in a strange new place. The room was dark, unfamiliar, and filled with noises he didn't recognize. But the moment I picked him up, he melted into me, his tiny body relaxing as he pressed his cheek against my chest. He didn't care about where we were. He only needed me—my warmth, my smell, my heartbeat. In that moment, I understood: I am his home.

Your embrace, your smell. Your snuggles and kisses. Your voice.

These are what home means to your baby. Wherever you are, there they are—in your memory, in your heart, in your arms. Around you, behind you, in front of you.

Today, take a moment to witness the impact you and your baby have on each other. Watch how their eyes light up when you smile, how their tiny hand searches for yours.

You are their first best friend. Their cheerleader and confidante. Their everything. And they, in turn, are your mirror—reflecting the purest love you've ever known.

You are their home, Mama.

Can you pause to feel the profound magic in this? The power of simply being *their* person. Because that's the kind of love that makes life beautiful.

(A PRAYER FOR TODAY)

May I remember that home is not a place, but the sacred space we create together, wherever we may be. In my embrace, we are grounded. In our connection, we are whole.

Sip of Self-Care:

Wear your baby in the carrier and set a timer for twenty minutes. You can even turn on your favorite music. Do a quick tidy up and light a candle for yourself. Not everything has to be in order but spending some time creating an inviting environment for you and your baby to enjoy is a form of self-love and self-care for you both.

The beauty of interdependence

There are millions of women all over the world who have taken this journey, something I find both soothing and enraging.

It soothes me because there is profound comfort knowing that I am not alone. There are others who have gone before me and have given it all they've got, and they've come out the other side a better version of themselves. It soothes me because I know that motherhood becomes easier when you have a village to lean on—a village that is yours, that sees you wholly for who you are as a woman *and* mother.

And yet, it enrages me because, as a culture, we have strayed so far from this wisdom. Instead of honoring the sacred web of interdependence, we celebrate "supermom syndrome" and glorify hyper-independence. In doing so, we've forgotten how to truly lean on each other, how to weave the kind of village that nurtures not just our babies, but us—*the mothers who are rising, stumbling, and growing alongside them.*

It takes a village to raise a child, yes—but it also takes a village to raise a mother.

Wherever you find yourself today, take a moment to soften. Let love in for yourself. Let the village in, as it is a tender refuge from the sometimes cold, harsh world. And if you don't yet have a support system, seek one—online, in person, wherever you are. Light a flare in the darkest of night and trust that the people who see your light will gather, ready to meet you in your need.

(A PRAYER FOR TODAY)

May my heart find peace and rest in knowing there are millions of women who have done this over and over again. I am capable. I am strong. I am enough. Desiring deeper support and connection doesn't make me weak, it makes me beautifully, powerfully human.

Repeat after me: I have everything I need

It is easy to get caught up in all the things you want, but if someone stopped you on the street today and asked you what you *need* right now, where you are lacking, you may have to ransack your brain a bit.

Recently, I stood in my kitchen, overwhelmed by the chaos of motherhood—dishes piled up, laundry spilling over, a baby on my hip. I felt the weight of wanting things to be smoother, easier. But then, my baby let out the tiniest laugh, and suddenly everything else melted away. That sound was a reminder: I already have what matters most. A home filled with love. A healthy little one. The strength to figure it all out.

On days when it feels like you wish you had more—more peace, more reassurance, more resources—look around you and take in the moments with your baby, your home, the support you do have, and the identity you are now carving for yourself as an emboldened mother, partner, woman, leader.

The truth is, you have everything you need, within you, around you. Can you feel it?

(A PRAYER FOR TODAY)

I have everything I need. I am grateful for everything that is mine and currently here, in my life, for me and my baby.

The anti-herd mentality

Not long ago, I was at the airport, rushing to make it through security. As I approached the checkpoint, I noticed a long line of people waiting in one lane. Everyone was standing there, shuffling forward inch by inch. I almost joined them without thinking, because if everyone else was in that line, it must be the right one, right?

But something made me pause. I glanced around and saw three other lanes, completely open, just a few steps away. No one was in them. Then it hit me—the crowd wasn't right, they were just following the person in front of them. And I had almost done the same.

This moment stuck with me because it's emblematic of the human condition. How often do we find ourselves standing in the same metaphorical line as everyone else, not because it's where we're meant to be but because it feels easier to follow the crowd than to pause, look up, and choose a path of our own?

Is the alignment you're walking in truly yours? Is it God's? Are those two in harmony—or are you following the pull of everyone else's expectations?

Do you make moves for yourself, your family, and your baby based on what is in alignment with you and in what works for all of you? Or are they shaped by the pressure to keep up, to please others, or to meet someone else's standards?

When we feel rushed, stressed, or disconnected, it's often because we've wandered from our center. Your path requires a deeper truth—your truth. Come back to your center, Mama. Come back to the voice within that whispers to you how insightful you are based on your own unique experiences. Come back to the mother's intuition within you that already knows what her baby needs.

Pause, look around, and choose the open lane that aligns with you. Deep breaths. Come home to you.

(A PRAYER FOR TODAY)

May I remember that it is safe to walk in alignment with my soul. It is safe to do what I feel is best for me, my baby, and my family.

The circle of care

Have you ever heard about how female elephants gather around when one of them gives birth? It's so beautiful. They form this protective circle, shielding her and her baby from anything that might come their way. They stand there, strong and steady, so she can focus on bonding with her little one. I can't stop thinking about how much that mirrors what we need as mothers.

Motherhood isn't meant to be done alone. We're meant to have our own herd—the women in our lives who just *get it*. Maybe it's your best friend who drops by with coffee and doesn't care that your house is a mess. Or your sister, who tells you you're doing an amazing job even when you feel like you're falling apart. Maybe it's your mom or grandmother, who show up with stories of their own early days and remind you that this phase is hard but fleeting. Or the mom friend from your baby group who texts you at 2 a.m. because she's awake too.

These women aren't just there for the little things—they're the lifeline you didn't even know you'd need. Like those elephants, they're standing guard around you, holding you steady when you feel unmoored. Their presence fills you up when your tank is running on fumes.

Let them in, Mama. Let them bring you meals, hold your baby, or just sit and listen when you need to cry. Lean into their support. It's how we were made to do this. We thrive when we let ourselves be held by our herd.

(A PRAYER FOR TODAY)

Bless the women in my circle: the ones who cheer me on, lift me up, and remind me of my strength. May we continue to hold and support one another.

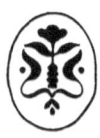

Sip of Self-Care:

Create Your Self-Care Menu

Take a moment to list all the activities that truly make you feel good. Write everything down, no matter how big or small. Then, divide your list into three categories based on how much time each activity takes:

- Under 5 Minutes: Quick resets, like deep breathing, stepping outside for fresh air, or lighting a candle.

- 5–10 Minutes: Slightly longer moments, like a short walk, journaling, or sipping tea mindfully.

- Over 10 Minutes: More immersive practices, like a bath, a yoga session, or reading a chapter of your favorite book.

Think of this as your personal self-care menu. Keep it somewhere visible and aim to choose at least one item from it each day, based on the time and energy you have. This menu becomes a gentle reminder that care for yourself is not a luxury, it's a practice. Even the smallest choice can shift your energy and bring you back to center.

Let love be your guiding light

You don't have to have it all figured out, Mama.

When I take a moment and reflect on motherhood, then recollect the experiences I had growing up, I view my mother with such deep compassion. Because she, too, was winging it, trusting her intuition, loving and raising us with her whole heart and soul. She didn't have it all figured out, she simply allowed herself to show up as she was—full of love. Love illuminated the path so she could see the next step ahead.

As children, we often see our parents as superheroes, infallible and all-knowing. But the truth is, they were figuring it out in real time, just as we are. They learned as they went, stumbling, growing, and evolving alongside us.

When I was growing up, my mom didn't have much help, yet she managed to get three little kids out the door every day. In her whirlwind of multitasking, she often perched me on the bathroom countertop while she hurriedly put on her makeup. What she may not realize is how sacred those moments were. Perched up there, I had a front-row seat to her world. I'd watch her, wide-eyed, as she brushed and blended, absorbing her every move with admiration. Those fleeting moments—etched in memory and captured in photos—weren't just routine, they were the quiet magic of connection.

The same is true for you and your baby. You don't have to have it all figured out and you won't. You simply have to show up with love. Love is your guiding light, the steady flame illuminating the next step. One moment, one day, one heartbeat at a time.

(A PRAYER FOR TODAY)

Give me the courage to approach the voyage of motherhood with patience, gentleness, grace, and compassion—toward myself and my baby. I don't need to know everything, I simply need to be here now.

Mother the mother

As you mother your child, remember to mother yourself too. You embody the feminine archetype of creation and connection, a force as ancient and vital as the earth itself. The feminine archetype is not simply about giving but about balance. It's an intimate dance between creation and restoration, between pouring out and filling up. Just as the sun's rays nurture the earth's soil, let self-love, compassion, and care permeate your being, creating a harmonious rhythm of replenishment that ripples through both your soul and that of your little one.

Recognize the profound interconnectedness of this cycle, where the love you show yourself resonates with the love you pour into your child, fostering a bond that echoes through generations.

You are not merely a mother; you are a living vessel of creation, worthy of the tenderness and grace you so effortlessly share with the world. Nurture yourself as you nurture life, for in doing so, you honor the sacred rhythm of motherhood itself.

(A PRAYER FOR TODAY)

God, may I remember the value you have placed on my life. You created me from my mother's womb and love me endlessly. Remind me to show myself kindness in each moment so I may model for my child what it looks like to love yourself fully.

The buzzing energy surrounds you

As human beings, we sometimes feel like we are the center of the universe, but really, we are merely a part of it. I want my baby to understand and connect to this idea/value deeply.

Everything is vibrating—can you see it?

Everything is speaking—can you hear it?

Everything is breathing—can you feel it?

From the abstract perspective, the epitome of this Spring season is an aliveness. There is a symphony of energies all around us if we choose to tune in. In the grind of everyday life, most of us miss it, like the subtle hum of a bumble bee that only comes into focus as we get closer, quieter.

As an intricate part of this, our energy also sends out ripples, impacting the frequency of the people, plants, animals, and things around us.

So, ask yourself—and explore with your baby—this question: How can we make an impact on the vibration of other things in our environment today?

A deeper connection to one another. A deeper connection to the earth. A deeper connection to your soul's purpose. A deeper connection to gratitude. A deeper connection to love.

Let your energy be your guide.

(A PRAYER FOR TODAY)

May my thoughts, words, and actions be steeped in devotion and love. May my life's imprint be one of joy.

Peace out, people pleaser

I'll be the first to admit: I've always been a "yes" gal.

Saying yes felt like a badge of honor—a sign that I was open, flexible, and ready for anything. But now? I'm rethinking that. The truth is, I can't do as many things as I used to in a day or a week when it was just my own time and energy I had to consider.

Motherhood has taught me to slow down—and maybe that's the lesson I was meant to learn all along. Our children have a way of inviting us to pause, to move with intention, and to value presence over productivity. Every single day we have to make a series of choices: What is the priority? How will we spend our energy? And every day is a fresh start. Over the past six months, I've had countless moments when I thought, *Okay, that was too much.* But instead of spiraling into guilt, I realized the beauty lies in *learning* from that experience. I can simply choose a different way next time.

So, here's what I'm asking myself, and maybe you need to ask yourself too:

- What boundaries do you need to put in place to protect your energy?
- Are you committing to too much?
- Are you letting others set the tone for your life?

(A PRAYER FOR TODAY)

Grant me the wisdom and strength to establish healthy boundaries in my life. Help me honor my needs and values and guide me in setting limits that nurture my well-being and relationships.

Sip of Self-Care:

The Power of Yes and No

This week, give yourself the gift of intentional boundaries. Decide how many times you'll say *no*—whether to a workout, a social invitation, or even a text that feels like too much. If you're someone who craves more exploration or connection, flip the script and set a number of times to say *yes*—to trying something new, stepping outside your comfort zone, or prioritizing what excites you.

Each intentional *yes* or *no* is a small but powerful step toward creating a life that feels more aligned, more purposeful, and more authentically yours. Remember, this practice isn't about perfection, it's about progress. Honor yourself in every decision.

EXTRA SIP:

Keep a mental or written note of your yeses and noes this week. Reflect on how each choice feels in your body and heart. Let this practice guide you toward a rhythm of living that nurtures your well-being.

Fluidity over force

Today, the intention I offer you is both simple and profound: to be like water.

Water flows effortlessly, slipping through fingers, yet possesses the strength to carry a ship across vast oceans. It doesn't resist; it adapts. It finds the openings, molds to its surroundings, and transforms the places it touches. Water teaches us that true strength isn't found in force but in *fluidity*, in surrendering to the path that naturally unfolds.

We can find the flow, the softness in so many different parts of our lives. Right now, I'm learning that rest is not a retreat but a sacred act of surrender. In rest, I loosen my grip on the illusion of control and open my heart to God's rhythm. It is my quiet way of saying, "I trust you." Trust in the rhythm of life, in divine design. Rest is the way I set down the burdens I was never meant to carry, a way of remembering that the weight of the world is not mine to hold.

Water never questions whether it can hold up the ship; it simply does—just by being. God has already taken care of the how. My part is to flow, to trust, to let go.

Rest allows me to embody the qualities of water—fluid but strong. In the stillness, I feel God's presence most deeply. Surrender is not weakness, it is strength wrapped in grace.

Today, repeat this mantra: "I flow. I rest. I trust."

(A PRAYER FOR TODAY)

Help me flow with grace and strength, trusting in your plan. As I rest, remind me that surrender is faith in action. Carry what I cannot, and let my heart align with your will today and always.

You are born whole and holy

As humans, we are born whole and holy. There is nothing more evident of this than the first time we hold our baby. No matter the circumstances sur- rounding birth, a baby emerges as pure perfection. It's truly an awe-inspiring experience impossible to describe. A being created by God defines us as holy, and we come equipped with everything needed within ourselves, making us whole. Yet we spend our entire lives questioning these things. We go on a lifelong hero's journey in search of completion, only to realize we've been complete all along. A question you will ask yourself in every single season of motherhood without a doubt is: "Am I doing enough?" Here is a gentle reminder that you are.

Some moments are messy, some are lovely. There are high highs and low lows. This is the human experience, but let your perfect baby remind you that you are perfect in all your humanness too.

You, too, are whole and holy.

(A PRAYER FOR TODAY)

God, allow me to recognize my innate completeness. Let me see myself as I see my baby.

The magic in the mundane

Every action you take yields something of meaning. You put a load of laundry in, and your clothes are cleaned. You take a contact nap with your baby, and you feel a little more rested. You make yourself a delicious lunch, and you feel nourished. Even a quick meal standing over the counter offers you the gift of time for something else in your busy day.

Your daily momentum and milestones will vary in every season of motherhood. As you approach eight months on this journey, you will find countless moments worthy of celebration. Yes, even the moments that make you feel like you're not doing enough, the moments that make you question who you are, and even the most mundane moments in your day—celebrate them all.

Did you manage to get dressed, feed your baby, and leave the house today? That's a triumph.

Did you make some fun meals at home and take care of yourself and the baby? Applaud the effort.

Did you go to work, pick up your baby from daycare, cook dinner, and do bath and bedtime? That is resilience in action.

Today, I encourage you to celebrate these micro moments and new beginnings. Celebrate who you are, celebrate the beautiful baby you have, and celebrate how far you have both come. Find the magic in the mundane and shine some light on it today.

(A PRAYER FOR TODAY)

God, give me the grace to celebrate the different textures, blessings, and moments that each day brings. No day was created to be the same, but what I know is that I can do great things with love, as I am, wherever I am.

You have nothing to prove to anyone

You have nothing to prove to anyone about anything—your pregnancy, your birth experience, your postpartum experience, or even how you choose to journey in motherhood and the numerous initiations it will take you through. You are on a sacred and personal journey, one that requires no justification or approval from anyone else.

There have been many times in motherhood-related conversations over the past nine months when I have felt the need to justify my choices, but the truth is, I don't.

There may be moments when you feel the pull to defend your choices or explain your way of doing things. But let me remind you: you don't have to. Motherhood isn't a debate, and your path doesn't require validation.

Be mindful not to become the mother who tries to convince others that your way is the right way. That need to prove—or persuade—comes from a place of insecurity, not wisdom. If you think you know the "right" answer in someone else's story, you probably haven't read the whole book.

This year, you've embarked on the single biggest mental, emotional, and physical feat of birthing a beautiful baby into the world. That alone is extraordinary. Let the projections slide off. Feel the softness and strength in your bones, the ferocity in your heart, the love and compassion within every part of you. Let that be your guiding light.

You have nothing to prove, Mama. You only need to be who you are called to be.

(A PRAYER FOR TODAY)

God, grant me strength and wisdom as I struggle with the feeling of needing to prove myself. Remind me of my inherent worth and your unconditional love in my life.

Sip of Self-Care:

Aligning with Your Heart's Vision

Take a quiet moment to center yourself and connect with your inner wisdom. Begin by lighting a candle or setting the tone with a few deep, intentional breaths. Then, with a journal or a blank piece of paper, write a list of your core values—the guiding principles that define who you are and what you stand for. Let these words flow freely, reflecting on what feels most important to you as a person, partner, and parent.

Next, craft a heart vision for yourself and your family. Envision the life you're nurturing—how it feels, the energy it holds, and the legacy you want to create. Write it out as if you're describing it to your future self, filled with love and intention.

As you hold this vision, commit to aligning your decisions and actions with these values. Choose to receive guidance and advice only from those whose lives resonate with your soul's truth. Trust your intuition—it is your most reliable compass.

Nourish the garden within

There are new seeds stirring in your heart, your mind, and your soul as you continue to nourish the abundance that is motherhood. These seeds need more than nourishment though, they need spaciousness to take root, to breathe, and to expand. The best ideas, life-changing moves, and growth often arise when we allow these seeds the room they need to flourish.

The garden of your home, your life, your mind and soul, and your relationships will require you to dig up the weeds regularly to make space for new roots to grow. This work takes discernment, the kind that comes with the courage to lean deeply into who you are called to be, here and now, in this phase in your life.

And remember, discernment thrives when you nourish yourself first. The garden of your soul requires tending—gentle care, quiet moments, and faith in the unseen growth that is unfolding before you.

(A PRAYER FOR TODAY)

God, guide me to nourish the garden of my soul. Give me the courage to be discerning of what and who is for me, my baby, and my family. And help me lovingly release everything that is no longer helping us grow.

You are worthy of honoring your needs

It's okay to ask for your space and to claim your peace.

Asking for your space may not always look like taking alone time to accomplish something. For a long time, I thought I needed an excuse to step away, hiding behind the task of pumping milk, just to carve out a moment for myself. I'd retreat upstairs, close the door, and exhale deeply. Sometimes I'd scroll on my phone or listen to a podcast while pumping—not because I had to, but because I craved a sliver of stillness. It took time to realize that I didn't need a reason or an excuse to take care of myself. I simply needed to ask. Sometimes you need space to simply be.

It can be space from your baby (yes, that's normal).It can be space from your family, friends, or the constant hum of the world (also normal). Asking for space doesn't have to be a confrontation or a declaration. It can be a quiet, steady reclamation—a soft yet resolute way of showing up for yourself. Without apology. Without shrinking. Without doubting the worth of your needs.

Motherhood can feel like the watering hole in the jungle, where everyone is coming to you to be replenished. But you need some of that good, fresh hydration for yourself. You can't pour endlessly from an empty vessel.

Reclaim that power, Mama, and ask for space when things feel like they're moving beyond your threshold.

You are worthy of care, worthy of space. You are worthy, always, in every way.

(A PRAYER FOR TODAY)

God, help me honor my need for rest without guilt and claim my space with grace. Fill me with your peace so I can give from the overflow of your love.

Surrender to the unfolding of your baby's personality

What are some beautiful traits you've noticed about your baby? During this season, they are continuing to develop their own quirks, personalities, and habits.

We can sometimes be quick to label our babies or let others label them. It can start as soon as the day they are born, shaping how we see them and how they grow. But here's an invitation to flip the script by finding the positive.

Reframing labels has become one of my passions (and a playful challenge). It's a way to see our little ones through a lens of possibility rather than limitation.

Instead of "Oh, he's a picky eater," try "He has refined tastes."

Rather than "She always wants to be held. She's going to become so dependent," say "She's so affectionate and loving."

Do you see where I'm going with this?

The labels we attach or allow others to attach to our baby now are the ones that stick subconsciously. Language is extremely powerful, and little minds absorb everything.

What if we allowed ourselves to surrender to the unfolding of our baby's developing personality without limitations or projections?

(A PRAYER FOR TODAY)

Let me view my baby as a beautiful blank canvas. May they grow into their uniqueness without any limitations, projections, or assumptions.

The frequencies of what surrounds you

Did you know that every *thing* on this planet carries a frequency too—a subtle energy that interacts with your baby's developing system? From the clothes they wear to the toys they hold, these items shape their sensory world in ways we often overlook.

Natural materials like wool, wood, and cotton resonate at higher frequencies that align with the body's natural vibrations. For example, linen and wool vibrate at approximately 5,000 Hz—much higher than the human body's average frequency of 100 Hz—potentially boosting energy and promoting well-being.

I once thought wooden toys and neutral palettes were just a minimalist trend. But I've come to see they represent something deeper: bringing the grounding essence of nature indoors. A wool blanket doesn't just warm your baby; it cradles them in the timeless energy of the earth. A wooden rattle isn't just a toy; it hums with the steady vibration of the tree it came from. These natural elements are alive with energy and connection.

That said, it's important to remember it doesn't have to be all or nothing. I have plastic items in my home, too, and they serve their purpose. This isn't about perfection or guilt, it's about starting to think intentionally about what you bring into your world.

The best part? You don't need to spend a fortune. Wool sweaters and cotton onesies can be found at thrift stores, wooden toys at secondhand shops, or you can even use repurposed items from your home.

Today, reflect on the items in your baby's world. Know that your intention in creating their environment infuses everything with love. And that love, more than any frequency, is what they'll feel most.

(A PRAYER FOR TODAY)

God, may I see the beauty in simplicity and honor the energy of natural things. Open my heart to find intention in the everyday, knowing that even the smallest choices can nurture a sense of peace and grounding.

Sip of Self-Care:

Spend five minutes today decluttering or swapping out one small thing in your space for something natural. Maybe it's replacing a synthetic air freshener with a sprig of eucalyptus or swapping a plastic cup for a ceramic mug. As you make this shift, notice how it feels to bring intention and care into your environment—not as a task, but as a quiet act of love for yourself and your baby.

Embracing the process of becoming

You are here, standing in the sacred chaos of new beginnings. You are growing, reshaping, and nurturing the life that was once a dream—a prayer carved into reality.

I think of Michelangelo, how he saw the sculpture already inside the block of stone. He didn't create David, he freed him. Maybe that's what this season is for you—chipping away, piece by piece, to reveal the truest, rawest version of yourself. You're not building something new, you're uncovering what's already there. Your baby, your matrescence, they are the chisel, breaking apart who you thought you had to be to reveal who you truly are.

Allow yourself to unfold deeper into this season.

This baby is a prayer answered, but that doesn't mean it's easy.

Part of your initiation into this new identity as a mother, woman, partner, friend is allowing yourself to fully feel it all. To stand in your power and know that the mess and the magic are both part of the masterpiece.

You are here, Mama. You have arrived (even if it doesn't always feel that way) and yet, you're still becoming. Trust the process, trust yourself, and let the beauty of this season remind you that the masterpiece was always within you. Motherhood is meant to uncover the deepest parts of you, if only you will let it.

(A PRAYER FOR TODAY)

Deepen my alignment in this powerful and sacred initiation of motherhood. What a blessed journey this is. I am grateful for every single prayer I am living out loud, here and now.

Honor the cyclical nature of all parts of life

Spring reminds us that the seeds we've planted in seasons past may be ready to bloom. It's a time of renewal and growth, and I want to remind you today that even if your life looks different from how it once did, you are not lost. You are simply walking a new path, one that is guiding you home to yourself in a deeper, more profound way.

I remember one evening, standing in the laundry room surrounded by piles of tiny clothes, feeling utterly invisible. It had been one of those long days—meals cooked, tears wiped, and endless bottles washed. I wondered, *Does any of this even matter? Do they notice?*

And then later that night, as I rocked my baby to sleep, I felt it. The way he melted into my chest, his breathing soft and steady, his little hand gripping my shirt. In that moment, I realized it all matters. The unseen work, the quiet care, the countless small acts of love—they are the foundation of my family's world.

Did you know that a mother's body doesn't just physically nourish her child, it also builds emotional safety? Studies show that a baby's sense of security comes largely from their connection to their caregiver, and those everyday acts of devotion—like feeding, cuddling, and simply being present—are what shape that bond.

Mama, your love is felt in every meal you prepare (or order), every bath given, every diaper changed, every snuggle shared. Even if no one says it, your family feels the warmth of your care in every moment. You are the oil that keeps the lamp burning, the salve that soothes, the light that brightens their days.

If today feels heavy, please remember you are appreciated in ways that words may never express. And you are truly amazing.

(A PRAYER FOR TODAY)

May I remember that I am whole. I am enough. I am love. I am courageous.

Now you know

Now you know a mother's love.

It is as fierce as a wolf, while being as sweet as a pot of honey.

It is more sacred than the rarest gem, more delicate than the finest piece of thread.

Now that you know a mother's love, there is no going back, no undoing. There is only forward momentum.

There are some things in life you can't possibly understand until you go through them yourself. Someone can describe them to you in a hundred different ways, but until you have that experience, it just doesn't click.

Motherhood is like that.

I am constantly late now, or making plans I can't keep, and I want to be around people who understand, who get it, or who are at least willing to try and show me compassion along the way. I often think of my friends who had kids before me. Did I show up for them like I should have? Sadly, probably not. I just didn't really know *how to* show up. Or those mothers on airline flights in my past who had a child kicking my seat or crying. I cringe now at my reaction because they were just doing their best (and were probably stressed themselves).

I didn't know then, but I know now.

So, I will live and respond differently. I will show up for my friends in a way I hope they will show up for me. I will hurry to open the door for a mother with a stroller as I head into the coffee shop. Better yet, I will buy her a coffee.

Let motherhood rearrange and change you and your way of showing up in the world.

Because once you know, you know.

(A PRAYER FOR TODAY)

Thank you for opening my eyes to the blessing of motherhood. As my heart softens, allow me to use my experience to love big and embody your spirit through my actions toward my family, friends, and others.

Impermanence is your permanence

The only constant in life is change: evolution, impermanence, growth.

No matter how you look at it, your permanence lies in accepting impermanence.

Conceiving your baby: impermanence.

Carrying your baby for the better part of a year, and the physical, emotional, hormonal, and mental changes that occur during pregnancy: impermanence.

Birthing your baby: impermanence.

Raising your baby and finding yourself in the transformation of matrescence: impermanence.

The way you show up differently for yourself, your relationships, your career, and your aspirations: impermanence.

While it might sound scary (and feel scary in the moments you're walking through it), impermanence is the most beautiful gift of life. You get to choose how you adapt, pivot, grow, evolve, show up, respond, love, and do things differently. You get to reinvent yourself at every turn, in every moment. Your resilience is strengthened.

The present is the only moment you have for certain. And love.

All else is impermanent, blessed change.

(A PRAYER FOR TODAY)

Help me lean into the constant that is change. May I approach each day with an open mind, body, heart, and spirit so that change and I can dance a beautiful tango.

Sip of Self-Care:

Write down (or mentally ponder) two to four things that you would like to be different right now. Maybe it's the agony of your baby teething or the guilt you feel when leaving for work. Then, next to those items, list how long it's been going on and how long you expect it to last. Notice that nothing is indefinite; rather, each item is temporary.

Your enoughness will shine through

Last night, as my baby's raspy cough broke the stillness, I rocked him in the glow of the humidifier, feeling completely drained. I hadn't slept, the laundry had taken on a life of its own, and my to-do list seemed like a distant dream. I wanted to cry, but instead, I held him closer.

In that quiet moment, I realized something: my enoughness wasn't in what I got done or how perfect my life looked. It was in the way I soothed him, the way I stayed present, even when I felt like I had nothing left to give. My love was enough.

And so today, I want to remind you too . . .

On days when it feels like your energy is nonexistent or you're on your proverbial last straw: *Your enoughness will carry you through.*

On days when it feels like nothing goes as planned, when your baby's needs take over, and when it feels like you're falling behind because you're trying to keep up with your idealized version of a new mom, please remember: *Your enoughness will guide you home.*

Back to your body.

Back to your breath.

Back to loving yourself, your baby, and your life in ways only you can, Mama.

(A PRAYER FOR TODAY)

Dear God, on days when I feel like the last drop of courage has left my spirit, or when my soul feels like it isn't enough, may I see myself in the way you see me. May I move in the ways you created me to be—whole, nourished, loving, graceful, and compassionate.

Motherhood is a bittersweet symphony

Some days you cannot help but smile at all the progress you're making in your motherhood journey, all the milestones your baby is bravely reaching, soaking in the love shared with those around you. On other days, it might feel monotonous, like the same scene playing over and over, leaving you longing for a spark of something new. Some days you'll stand tall, bursting with pride at the strength you showed through pregnancy, birth, and postpartum. Other days, your inner lioness will want to roar out loud for all the ways in which your experience hasn't been validated or honored.

Wherever you find yourself, honor that space.

Motherhood isn't easy. It has many tunes. Some harmonize well; others are a deafening screech. It's a bittersweet symphony.

Honor the off-beaten path, Mama. It's the beat of your soul that will keep this symphony going, even when the world seems silent, and that is something extraordinary.

(A PRAYER FOR TODAY)

May the heartbeat of my soul forever guide me home on this journey of motherhood.

A note on creativity

While you're in this fertile initiation exploring the divinity of mother energy, wise woman power, and the sacred heart, this entry invites you to fully embrace your creative potential. Let inspiration flow freely to help move the stuck energy of the routine of everyday life.

Paint. Experiment with new recipes. Complete a project with your partner or loved ones. Write. Create.

Record your voice for your baby. Film their milestones. Make a baby journal in which you write to them weekly (or however often your heart desires). Buy a polaroid or disposable camera so you can feel the prints in your hand.

Explore new friendships. New spaces. New outfits. New hairstyles.

Don't think of yourself as an artist? Look at your baby—that little human is the best creative project you have co-designed with God. So, go confidently in the direction that fuels you and your creative heart.

Go in the spaces that bring you peace and comfort, and in those that make you feel wholly seen for who you are as you continue to evolve and morph into the most powerful version of yourself yet.

In this stage of motherhood, we have deeper access to the feminine that harnesses our creative energy, so use it and see what magic unfolds.

Fuel your creativity in any way you can.

(A PRAYER FOR TODAY)

Bless each day of mine with creativity. May it be a nourishing gift for my soul, my baby, and all those around me.

The most divine control lies in letting go

One thing I know for sure is that if we could control everything (and I mean *everything*), we would!

Before becoming a mother, I lived under the comforting illusion of control. Then pregnancy, birth, and motherhood arrived, shattering that notion and leaving me spinning. We think that if we plan enough or read enough or buy enough, we can control the outcomes.

Can you blame us?

There is so much that falls on us as mothers. Every decision sends some cascading effect on our child beginning the moment we discover we are growing human life within our body. It can be heavy.

Yet, the most sacred control lies in letting go.

Still, there are *parts* of an experience you can control, such as your responses, your words, your thoughts, and your receptivity to change. In essence, you can control your side of things. And then there are things you simply cannot control, including how your body responds in a critical moment, the type of emergency care you or baby may have needed in birth, your career circumstances or internal politics, the dynamics in relationships, and the temperament of your baby.

There is a limit to our control that can feel like a curse. But I want to remind you today that it can also be a blessing.

All those things you can't control? Hand it over to God. Truly, give it to God and let it unfold how it is meant to. You don't have to do it all, Mama. You can release your grip on it all, knowing that you won't fall while being carried by the spirit working *for you* in this life.

(A PRAYER FOR TODAY)

Dear God, teach me to surrender into your divine alignment and timing.

Sip of Self-Care:

The Worry Jar: Letting Go with Intention

Create a "worry jar" or "worry box" in your house to help externalize your worries. Write your worries on a sticky note and drop it in the jar. Visualize yourself giving it over to God. It is officially out of your hands.

This practice can give you a sense of control over your worries (you have done something with them—i.e., handed them over to a greater power) without allowing them to overwhelm you.

A note on capturing the moment

Capture it all, Mama. For you, for them, for the legacy they will most definitely be curious about as they grow older.

There is no such thing as too many memories captured on camera.

Think back to your childhood—who took most of the pictures?

Think back to if there were more pictures of you with your mom. How would that make you feel? Don't hesitate to ask someone to capture you and your baby. And on days when there's nobody to ask, do some selfie shoots with them.

Document the firsts, the little moments, and the big days—not for social media (unless that's your thing), but for your soul so you can remember yourself in this exact moment.

Record your baby's voice, their expressions, their slurps, their raspberry kisses, and their giggles.

I assure you, these memories will come in handy when you're feeling nostalgic for these moments, which you inevitably will.

(A PRAYER FOR TODAY)

May every moment I capture be raw and filled with grace and love and unfiltered joy. Teach me to see the beauty in each moment.

A nourished nervous system

Today, check in with your nervous system. Notice your breath. Is it shallow and hurried, as if rushing to keep up? Or is it grounded and steady, flowing deeply into your being?

Notice your posture. Are your shoulders scrunched up to your ears, bracing for impact? Or are they soft and aligned, an open invitation to ease?

Notice your facial tightness. Is your jaw clenched, holding unspoken words or tension? Or is it relaxed, free to smile, sigh, or express yourself fully?

Notice your belly. Does it feel wound up, a storm of emotions crashing within? Or does it feel relaxed, non-turbulent, and rooted?

Take a moment to scan your entire body each day. Notice where you're holding onto tightness, tension, grief, guilt, shame, frustration, and sadness. Notice where you feel ease, peace, and wholeness flowing through. Now, reflect on the balance between your sympathetic and parasympathetic states.

Your sympathetic nervous system is your body's "fight-or-flight" mode. It's the surge of energy that helps you respond to stress or demands, the spark that readies you for action. It can feel like a racing heart, shallow breath, tight muscles, or a flood of thoughts clamoring for attention. It's essential for survival but not meant to dominate every moment. Your parasympathetic nervous system, on the other hand, is your "rest-and-digest" mode. It's the soft hum of relaxation that allows your body to heal, your mind to center, and your spirit to feel safe. It shows up in slow, steady breaths, a calm heartbeat, and a sense of ease. It's where growth, connection, and restoration flourish. These two states are meant to work together to keep you balanced. But in the rhythm of motherhood—with its demands, joys, and surprises—it's easy to get stuck in overdrive when living in the sympathetic state too long.

Breathe deeply. Inhale love, grace, and compassion and send them to every part of yourself. A regulated nervous system is the foundation needed to thrive. Take time to nourish it and breathe life into yours, then bring it into balance again and again.

(A PRAYER FOR TODAY)

May I nourish my nervous system daily with loving kindness and compassion.

Mothers rock

Before birth, we are the rock star—both the rock and star. The steady force growing life within us, and the radiant centerpiece everyone celebrates. People gather to honor us, to marvel at the glow of pregnancy, to revel in the miracle we're carrying. Partners look at us with awe, as if we're holding the universe itself. For those fleeting months, we are everything—the anchor and the light, the gravity and the glow.

But after birth, the balance shifts. In an instant, the baby becomes the star, shining brilliantly at the center of every moment. The world's gaze moves to them—their tiny hands, their coos, their cries, their every milestone. Visitors bring gifts for the baby, ask about the baby, adore the baby. And we, the mother, sometimes quietly fade into the background. While our bodies, minds, and hearts are healing from the most profound transformation, we can feel like we've been cast in a supporting role. No longer the star, we become the rock—the steadfast foundation holding it all together.

It's beautiful and humbling . . . and hard. To go from being both the rock and the star to just the rock can feel disorienting. But Mama, remember even the brightest star needs something unshakable to orbit around, something strong to keep them steady. That's you. You are the gravity, the strength, the quiet power that makes it all possible.

Here's the truth: In the story of *your* life, you are still the main character. As you pour yourself into your child, don't lose sight of your own worth. Your dreams, your joys, and your struggles still deserve center stage. You are not just the rock holding up someone else's world, you are the star illuminating your own. Keep that truth close. You are still the hero of this story—even if the spotlight now dances on the one you love most.

(A PRAYER FOR TODAY)

Thank you, God, for allowing me to shine strong and bright for my beautiful new star and remember my innate worth and light. Remind me that my strength and presence are not diminished but magnified in this sacred season of motherhood.

Creating traditions

In the world you envision for yourself, your baby, and your growing family . . .

Who will you become?

What will you be doing? What moments fill your day?

What values do you want to impart on your child as they grow?

What traditions do you want to incorporate into your family's story? Ones that are new or ones that are passed down from your own childhood?

Here is a glimpse of a tradition I'm dreaming up. Each year for my son's birthday, we'll choose a song lyric as the theme and then sing that song at the party. We'll even print the lyrics so everyone feels welcomed to join in on the singing. His first birthday can be "What a *one*-derful world"; his second, "Fly me *two* the moon," and so on. My father-in-law loves to sing, so I'll put him in charge of leading us in the theme songs. We plan to capture my son's grandpa singing his heart out on a yearly basis. I want my son to have that memory.

What do you want to create or invite into your little one's world? What rituals will make your days sweeter, more meaningful, and full of connection? The time passes so quickly, but when we pour intention into the small moments, they take on a glow of nostalgia and become the foundation of something timeless.

(A PRAYER FOR TODAY)

May we become a pure channel of love, peace, comfort, and joy everywhere we go, in all that we do, in all that we are, in all that we are becoming.

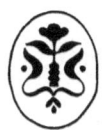

Sip of Self-Care:

Write a family manifesto for yourself, your partner, and your baby. Place it somewhere where you can see it daily. Let this be a place of inspiration from which the traditions of your family flow.

Let go and let God

Surrender doesn't mean giving up, it means letting up on the *resistance*. What are you surrendering to God at this moment? Let yourself lean into it, wholly.

Surrender your expectations for your baby and their growth and development, embracing the unfolding journey. Surrender your body and health, and the sacred transformation of your soul as she evolves. Surrender your marriage or partnership, trusting in love's ability to withstand and adapt. Surrender your career aspirations and desires and the need to control your outcome. Pause your resistance to the present. Relish where you are currently placed, *right now*. Surrender with the tension in strained family and friend relationships. Surrender deeply with your whole being all that feels too much, too soon.

Sometimes you just have to let go and let God. You don't need to navigate this season in isolation. Lean on your support systems; but more importantly, lean into God. All you have to do is stay open to receive, ask for whatever it is you most need, then surrender the rest.

At the end of the day, I envision gathering all my to-dos, worries, and unanswered questions and placing them on God's altar. I visualize each burden being lifted from my shoulders, one by one, until I feel lighter, from head to toe. My mind softens, my heart expands, and I allow myself to rest deeply, knowing that my worries and plans are in the safest hands—God's hands. This practice doesn't just ease my body, it fills me with peace and opens me to receive what I need for tomorrow.

Whenever you feel the weight of your day pulling you down, try this. Let it go, and let God carry it for you. Peace comes from letting anything that is not directly in your control to be out of your mind as well. Rest, knowing you are held.

(A PRAYER FOR TODAY)

Guide me to surrender anything that feels heavy, uncertain, uncomfortable, or challenging. Let me always remember that you walk with me in each moment, God. I am not walking this hill alone.

A note on forgiveness and compassion

Forgiveness isn't weakness, and compassion isn't a vulnerability—they are your quiet superpowers, especially as a mother.

Like sunlight to a plant, these acts of grace fuel your growth, transforming the hard moments into something life-giving. When cultivated daily—for yourself, your baby, and your loved ones—forgiveness and compassion work like photosynthesis, turning the raw energy of love and struggle into strength and resilience.

Forgive yourself for the moments you lost your cool, felt flustered, or didn't meet your own expectations.

Forgive yourself for the moments you thought you had to do things a certain way because "that's how it's always been done."

Forgive yourself for being too hard on your body, your emotions, your heart, for all the times you felt "not enough."

Forgive yourself for carrying the weight of others' emotions, projections, and limitations, even when it wasn't yours to bear.

Have compassion for the version of yourself that you were before you started the adventure of motherhood. She didn't know what was to come.

Have compassion for the woman you were before motherhood. She didn't know what was coming, and yet she stepped into the unknown with courage. Forgive her for tolerating behaviors that crossed her boundaries, for bending and breaking to meet expectations that no longer fit. Forgive her for feeling the need to explain her choices—how she parents, loves, or navigates the sacred transitions of pregnancy, birth, and postpartum. Inhale compassion, exhale forgiveness—for all, yourself included.

(A PRAYER FOR TODAY)

May I continue to extend forgiveness and compassion toward myself, my baby, my loved ones, and anyone else who needs it. I release all old stories and circumstances. I forgive myself and others for not knowing then what we know now. Guide me as I move forward with grace.

Prioritize what matters most to you now

It's okay to reorganize your priorities.

Exhale a deep breath if you need that reminder today! I know I do.

At first, feelings of guilt can surface as you juggle two lives: the one you had before the baby arrived, and the one you are currently living as a mother. Over time, however, these feelings will dissipate as you realize it's safe for your priorities to shift based on this season of life.

Weeknight dinner and drinks with colleagues or friends may have now turned into precious family time together. Or perhaps you once felt called to move away from extended family, but now you yearn to be close.

Solo, carefree weekends have now turned into days for running errands timed with your baby's nap schedule. Maybe you're now cozying up at home, or exploring places with each other and your baby, or having visits from family and friends.

Just know that it's okay to reorganize your priorities on this journey of motherhood, because as you evolve, so will those priorities.

(A PRAYER FOR TODAY)

God, help me honor what is being asked of me in this phase of my life and motherhood without any shame, guilt, or explanation.

Measure each day not by the fruits it yields,
but by the seeds you plant along the way

Motherhood is a portal for the blooming of your innermost dreams while healing your inner child. It's where you can play and express who you are in your deepest and fullest expression. This is where you can choose to nurture the most fruitful seeds.

What are some seeds, dreams, ideas you want to plant in your heart and your head—where they have the best chance of blooming?

For me, it was this book. I had the smallest inkling of an idea in the shower one day, and I let it marinate in my soul for some time (it was like I bought a pack of seeds but hadn't really figured out where to plant them yet). I shared my idea with a friend who connected me with a book doula who could help bring it to life. I gushed to my partner about how much I would love to work with her, and as it turns out, my first Mother's Day gift from him was a package with her. The rest is, as they say, history. It took root in my heart and from there blossomed in a way I never thought possible.

It is not our job to worry about the bloom—all we need to do is take the first step and plant the seed.

Honor your becoming in whatever speed that takes.

(A PRAYER FOR TODAY)

May I water the seeds I have planted with love, creativity, and excitement, and let me surrender to their blooming in your time, God, not mine.

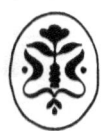

Sip of Self-Care:

Today, while you are changing your little one's diaper, try describing to your baby each step you take. Use uplifting phrases like "we are going to put a clean, fresh diaper on your sweet tush so you can be more comfortable." It may feel strange at first, but this narration is helpful for your baby to hear and ensures you are entirely present for the activity.

Capture the evolution

There was a time when I felt guilty about having my phone out, snapping photos of myself and my baby. Before I became a mother, I never took this many pictures of myself—it felt unnecessary, maybe even superficial. But now, when I scroll through the photos I've taken since his birth, I see them differently. Each one tells a story not just of how he's changed but of how I've changed too.

If you knew me five years ago, you probably wouldn't recognize the person I've become today. Motherhood has shifted me, pulled me, and reshaped me into someone new. Because we're immersed in the process, we don't always see the small ways we're growing day by day. But when I look back at these images, I marvel at the transformation, both his and mine.

We can't rely on memory alone to hold on to everything. How lucky are we to have these little time machines in our hands? A photographer friend once told me, "It only takes three seconds to capture a moment." That simple truth stuck with me.

So, take the picture, Mama. Bonus points if you're in it, because it's not just about recording their milestones, it's about documenting your evolution too. You don't have to look at it today, but save it for another day—when you need to remember just how far you've come. These images aren't just snapshots, they're evidence of the way you've bloomed, changed, and grown.

(A PRAYER FOR TODAY)

Thank you for the moments I get to hold in my hands and tuck away in my heart. What a gift it is to witness my baby's growth and my own. Help me see the beauty in my journey and the love that shines in me, even when I don't see it in the mirror. May every captured moment be a celebration of the transformation unfolding within me.

A note on mom guilt

One of the interesting things about mom guilt is that it has no real productive purpose.

Typically, when we feel "regular" guilt in other parts of our lives, it's often because deep down we know we shouldn't be doing what we're doing, whether it's eating that scoop of ice cream right before bed or gossiping about a friend. Guilt acts as our conscience.

But mom guilt is different. We feel it *even* when we are doing things well. We feel it when we are lying with our baby in the morning, cuddling and staring into their sweet eyes, and that gut-wrenching feeling arises that we should already be out of the house at a park enjoying the sunshine. What's the purpose of this feeling?

It sets in to paralyze us by making us believe that our perceived shortcomings are going to somehow mess up our children. It nags us into believing we aren't doing enough. When we lean into the mom guilt, it's often because we're comparing ourselves to others.

And now there is deep dissonance within us—with what our soul truly feels and how we show up versus how we are conditioned to show up for ourselves, our baby, and our family.

So today, if there is even a speck of mom guilt surfacing, don't brush it away. Instead, I want you to acknowledge it. Get curious.

Hmm, funny you're here. What are you trying to show me? Where did you first originate? Is there truth to this story you are telling me? Or is there an alternative version?

Notice your answers. Honor the truth that you excavate. Motherhood doesn't have to be inextricably intertwined with the feeling of guilt.

(A PRAYER FOR TODAY)

Help me release the guilt and shame that was never mine to carry or hold.

Motherhood as an offering

In some moments, motherhood can seem like a sacrifice. You have to let go of time, sleep, freedom, and fragments of the person you once were. But what if we saw it instead as a sacred offering to your family . . . and to the world. This offering is nothing short of extraordinary: your love, your energy, your unwavering presence. It's the raw, deliberate choice to pour yourself into love, moment by moment, day by day.

Every ounce of effort, every sleepless night, every whispered "I'm here." When you listen, when you hold, when you choose to be present despite the world trying to pull you in every direction. It all matters. Your love shapes your child, transforms you, and ripples outward in ways you'll never fully realize. This offering? It's unforgettable—woven into the hearts of those you love and the world you're shaping.

So, feel proud of yourself, Mama.

For navigating through each passing day with bravery, even when the path is unmarked.

For facing the many unknowns that come with this journey with a heart wide open.

For nourishing yourself, your baby, and your loved ones, in only ways you can.

For all the late nights and early mornings you've spent awake tending to, caring for, and nurturing your baby.

For showing up with fierce devotion in your matrescence journey.

Breathe deep, keep going, and trust in your strength. Your offering to the world is undeniably remarkable.

(A PRAYER FOR TODAY)

On days when I may not see how my love impacts those around me, may I remember that this comes from the source of life itself—God. Remind me that you are here, guiding, sustaining, and making my love matter in ways I may not yet understand.

How lovely is the silence of growing things

Growth isn't loud or obvious. It's not like a balloon expanding, where the change is in plain view. It happens when no one is watching. It happens in the spaces you can't see—deep within.

You may not even be aware of how this season of motherhood is shaping you, but you're becoming more confident in your role as a mother. You're learning to trust your instincts and are strengthening your footing in your matrescence journey.

When you have moments of doubt (and you will, which is normal), please be gentle with yourself. Take a few moments to remember just how far you've come. Think back to your first few weeks with your baby and take pride in the growth you've experienced as a woman, as a mother.

Pause, reflect, and give thanks to every messy, beautiful thing that has brought you here to this exact moment. It all counts. It has shaped you to be who you are: the mother your baby needs.

You've brought a life from the unseen realm to the seen. The world may not see the quiet strength it takes to rise over and over again as a mother. But those unseen efforts—those small, quiet acts—are the roots of something extraordinary.

You are doing an incredible job. Take a deep breath, trust in yourself, and know that you're laying a foundation for beauty and love to blossom. You're growing every day, in every moment. And unlike a balloon, *your* growth is limitless, boundless, infinite.

(A PRAYER FOR TODAY)

Thank you for every single moment that has led me here. Thank you for every single experience that has helped shape me into the person I am today.

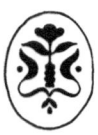

Sip of Self-Care:

Planting the Seeds of Inspiration

Set a timer for five minutes and grab a journal or a blank sheet of paper. Let your mind wander freely and jot down every idea or dream that excites you, big or small. Don't censor yourself—this is your creative space to explore. Whether it's something you've always wanted to try, a place you dream of visiting, or a goal you'd love to achieve, let it flow.

Once the timer goes off, take a moment to scan your list. Put a star next to the ideas that truly light you up—the ones that make your heart beat a little faster or fill you with joy.

Now, choose one or two of your starred ideas and create a simple, achievable action plan. Write down the first small steps you can take to bring these dreams to life. Maybe it's researching, setting aside time, or reaching out to someone who can guide you. Keep the steps manageable and realistic—it doesn't matter if they're for next week, next year, or five years from now.

The magic is in planting these seeds and trusting that, when the time is right, they will bloom beautifully. Let this practice remind you that nurturing your interests is a vital part of your journey.

Have faith

Your instinct as a mother is as innate and natural as breathing. This ancient technology is etched into your being, a divine compass guiding you toward what your child needs most. Have faith in it.

We have faith in God to guide us. We have faith in our loved ones to support us. But how many of us have faith in ourselves, especially when we're new to motherhood and learning as we go? If you're like me, you sometimes feel the pangs of self-doubt, questioning your actions, your instincts. As new moms, we want the absolute best for our baby and worry that we're not measuring up. But over these many months, I'm learning that I can believe in myself, and I hope you are too.

Just as you marvel at the beauty of nature and think of God, look at the beauty of your baby and feel assured that you're doing a great job—they are safe, happy, and loved. You can read your baby's expressions, their moods, their cries, and their coos. You were chosen by God, who knows you and values you. I was reminded of this recently during savasana in a yoga class. As the sun kissed my face through the window, it felt like a message—a gentle reminder that God is always *within* us, as steady and unwavering as the rising sun. When I was younger, I struggled with the idea of God "speaking" to us. I imagined booming voices and angels resembling something out of a cartoon. Now, I understand it differently. God's messages are subtle- felt in moments of quiet, in flashes of clarity, and in the whispers of our hearts. They're always there if we're willing to notice. Your instincts are one of those messages. They are a powerful language of love, attuning you to your baby's needs, emotions, and rhythms. Even when you feel uncertain about what to do next, they nudge you forward, an invisible guide showing you the way. Your instincts also warn you when something is off. They read the unspoken energy of people and situations. Some days your instincts may come as a soft whisper; other times, as a gut reaction or a roar. However they appear, trust them. These instincts are love letters from God, reminders of why you were chosen for your child. Have faith in the wonderful work you're doing for your little one. They certainly have faith in you.

(A PRAYER FOR TODAY)

May I learn to trust my intuition and instincts and have faith in myself as the wonderful mother you entrusted me to be for my baby.

What is the current soundtrack of your life?

Music has the power to heal, soothe, calm, activate, inspire, and excite, no matter the chaos that swirls around us. It helps us to express the inexpressible.

Go into your music app. What are some tracks you've been listening to on repeat? They can make you appreciative and nostalgic for a certain time in your life.

Do you sing any of these songs to your baby? I have never thought of myself as being musically inclined, but I love trying out new sounds and vocal tones with my son.

To your baby, there really is nothing sweeter than your voice.

A mother's singing is a celestial harmony that cradles their spirit and fills their world with tender light. So, I encourage you to pick a melody. Look up the lyrics and give it a whirl; they read like poetry.

It's uncanny the memory your child has and will continue to develop—most babies love the songs they listen to during this period. It's no coincidence that my son finds the Lumineers to be oddly soothing as he was listening to their album nonstop in the womb.

Today, for pure joy and fun, curate a playlist for you and your baby—one that soothes, one you can move and groove to, or one that allows you to relax and mellow out. It's a game changer, I promise.

(A PRAYER FOR TODAY)

May I approach every moment of this beautiful and powerful journey much like a musical journey. May I sing and dance and relax and rest in the moments that call for it.

Embrace the grace

It was one of those chaotic days—crumbs on the floor, toys everywhere, dishes stacked high. My husband, whose love language is acts of service, was quietly tidying up, wiping counters, folding laundry. After finishing the dishes, he turned to me and asked, "What more can I do?"

I paused, the weight of everything heavy on my heart. "Grace," I whispered. "I just need grace."

Grace—a gift of kindness we don't have to earn. It's the quiet permission to be human, to let go of perfection. It isn't about fixing everything; it's about embracing the beauty of what already is.

In that moment, I realized grace wasn't just for me, it was for all of us. For him, for me, for the baby giggling in the next room. Grace was the thread weaving love through our messy, imperfect life.

As you embrace the messiness that comes with this journey, let grace guide your ways like little roots spanning out in all directions to seek the hidden streams of strength within you.

Because it was never meant to be perfect. It was meant to be wholly *you*.

Not staged or perfectly sterile, but filled with love, messy imperfect perfection in all its glory.

So, give yourself grace more days than not. For you and your baby. For everything that competes for your attention and energy and capacity.

May grace be with you in every moment, wherever you go, wherever you are, and in whichever way you choose to show up.

(A PRAYER FOR TODAY)

I am gracefully finding myself as the loving, kind, patient, devoted, and present woman that I am.

The meditative mind

As a meditation guide, I've led hundreds of sessions for others, and one of the most common misconceptions I hear is that meditation requires a lot of preparation—a special time, a cushion, or even a completely clear mind. I'm here to remind you that none of that is necessary.

Meditation is simply about building a relationship with your awareness. It's not about silencing your thoughts but noticing *when* your attention drifts into the stream of thoughts—up to 70,000 a day—and gently guiding it back to the present moment.

Meditation is as simple as approaching any activity with full presence. Perhaps, right now that means cleaning bottles or giving your baby a bath. To harness the meditative mind, simply bring awareness to whatever it is you are doing.

When your mind inevitably wanders (because it will), that's not failure—it's an opportunity. Every time you bring your awareness back to the now, you strengthen your ability to meet life as it is rather than getting swept away by what was or what might be.

This naturally calms the nervous system and brings a sense of insight that can't come when our brains are busy ruminating over what happened or predicting what's to come. Meditation doesn't require perfection, only your willingness to return to what is directly in front of you.

(A PRAYER FOR TODAY)

God, bring me into meditative awareness so I find calm in the current moment.

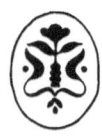

Sip of Self-Care:

A Mindful Stroll: Connecting with Your Baby and the World Around You

Take your baby out for a walk, leaving behind the noise of books, podcasts, or distractions. This is a time to be fully present. As you move, allow yourself to simply *observe*.

Notice the colors and textures of the world around you—the way the leaves flutter in the breeze, the patterns of sunlight on the path, or the gentle sway of trees. Listen to the sounds around you: birds chirping, the rustling of leaves, or even the soft coos or breaths of your baby.

Feel the rhythm of your steps and the connection between you and your little one. Let this moment anchor you in the here and now, shifting your focus from doing to simply *being*. Each step is an invitation to deepen your awareness and savor the beauty of presence.

Discover your seed incident

Have you ever heard the term "seed incident"? It's a concept coined by creativity researchers, and I think of it quite often these days. A seed incident refers to a seemingly small moment, an event or an experience, that quietly marks the beginning of something much bigger—a transformation, development, or realization.

The term is so fitting because, like a seed, these moments pack the potential for something much more impactful than what meets the eye. These incidents may feel ordinary or go unnoticed at first, yet they have the power to profoundly change our lives.

We often expect monumental shifts to announce themselves loudly, to look or feel significant from the start. But that's rarely how it works. Maybe it's the kind comment you gave to the person in the grocery line who then became your new mom friend. Maybe it's the time that you got lost on a walk with your baby and stumbled on your new favorite route. It could be a conversation with your employer about shifting into more manageable hours, and their unexpectedly supportive response planted a new sense of balance. Or the email you'd been scared to send that, once written, set something in motion.

The magical thing about the seed incident is its subtle. So, what does this mean for us in motherhood?

It's simple: Stay open—open to asking the questions, making the connections, forming new relationships. From there, the seed grows on its own fertile journey, expanding in ways you couldn't have predicted.

Take a moment to discover your own seed incident. Let it grow and allow its miracle to surprise you.

(A PRAYER FOR TODAY)

Guide me to be open to the seeds I am co-planting with God all around my life. Allow my heart and mind to expand in order to receive the blessings meant for me. May I feel safe unclenching my grip on growth.

Mind the motherhood speed limit

I used to be able to grab my keys and go. In fact, I prided myself on being able to squeeze the most out of a day. And then I became a mother.

I had a date with a friend yesterday and mapped the drive to be about fifteen minutes. I got my baby packed up, then fed him so he would be content for the drive (I hoped anyway—the car seat has always been a hit or miss for us in terms of him liking it).

All seemed well, and I grabbed my keys and the diaper bag with fifteen minutes to go. As we were walking out the door, I felt it: a large rumble through his tummy. And then . . . yep, you guessed it. Everywhere.

His whole outfit had to be changed. Mine did too. I felt frazzled and anxious. Honestly, I no longer wanted to meet my friend at that point.

Twenty minutes later, we finally crossed the threshold of the door yet again. I let the sun hit my face and took a deep, audible breath. I closed my eyes. I realized then that it had been the expectation of "perfect timing" that had made me feel anxious. In reality, being fifteen, thirty, even sixty minutes late wouldn't have been a big deal.

If we can let go of expectations and instead anticipate that delays may occur, it will be less jarring when they do happen.

The antidote to my anxiety wasn't in rushing, it was in surrendering. Motherhood doesn't curse us with chaos, it teaches us to embrace it. Our children aren't here to fit neatly into schedules. They're here to slow us down, to soften the sharp edges of our expectations, to build in us a resilience we didn't know we needed. It's up to us to let them.

(A PRAYER FOR TODAY)

May I surrender to the pace of my child instead of expecting them to keep up with my unrealistic one. Let me feel peace in moving slowly about my day so that my heart can remember the micro moments in the spaces in between.

Leading by example

I'll never forget the first time I felt the pang of guilt for choosing myself. My baby was still so little, and I had signed up for a two-day online breathwork certification course—a decision I'd agonized over for weeks. As the start time approached, I found myself wondering: *What kind of mother takes two full days to focus on herself while her baby is right there needing her?*

But I also knew how depleted I felt. I was running on fumes; I was overwhelmed and disconnected from myself. I knew I couldn't show up fully for my baby if I didn't take this time to refill my own cup. So, I set up everything my husband would need to care for our little one, closed the door, and logged on.

Those two days changed everything. Between the guided breathwork and intentional moments of reflection, I released emotions I hadn't realized I was holding on to. I felt a reconnection to myself that had been missing for months. And when the seminar ended, I opened the door, scooped up my baby, and felt something I hadn't in a long time: energized, grounded, and alive.

We're taught to believe that choosing ourselves—our needs, dreams, or even a moment of stillness—is selfish, especially in motherhood. But the truth is, you are the foundation of your family. Without you, there is no stability, no nourishment, no direction. Taking time to nurture yourself doesn't detract from your role as a mother, it fortifies it.

When you tend to your own well-being, you're not just doing it for yourself, you're doing it for your child. You're teaching them the value of self-care and balance, and you're creating a loving, stable environment where everyone can thrive. You can take care of others and of yourself. Be the example you want to set for your baby.

(A PRAYER FOR TODAY)

Remind me that when I go first, all else follows in pure alignment. Choosing myself is an integral part of my mental, emotional, physical, and spiritual alignment.

The alchemy you create

I've never met a single mother whose choices aligned perfectly with mine—and that's the beauty of it. That's the freedom.

There's no single path, no perfect way. The magic is in the way you listen to your heart, in the way you honor your instincts, and in the way you trust yourself to create a motherhood that reflects you and your baby. It gets to be your way, Mama.

The alchemy you create—unique, potent, and entirely your own—flows through every choice you make.

The way you show up for your baby.

The way you show up in your business or your career.

The way you slow down or speed up.

The way you choose to nurture your baby and yourself.

The way you choose to spend your time and who you choose to spend it with.

The way you connect with your baby.

The way you choose to express yourself.

It all gets to be done in alignment with who you are and who you are becoming on this beautiful journey of motherhood.

You are the love that turns the ordinary into the extraordinary. Let it be yours, and let it be enough.

(A PRAYER FOR TODAY)

May I continue to walk in alignment, no matter what.

Sip of Self-Care:

Explore the New in the Familiar

Take a walk today in a direction you haven't gone before. As you step outside, leave behind the familiar and embrace the unknown. Pay attention to the details around you—the unique houses, the sway of the trees, the sounds of footsteps or conversations nearby.

With each step, allow your senses to awaken. Notice what you might have overlooked in your usual routine—the colors, the textures, the patterns. Let this walk be a reminder that even the smallest changes can offer new perspectives, both in your surroundings and within yourself.

If you can, take a moment to pause, close your eyes, and take a few deep breaths. Let the stillness of the new path ground you, helping you feel present and open to the world around you. This simple shift can refresh your mind, body, and spirit.

You are more than you know

You are the light of your baby's life. Their everything.

You are the hope in your family's life.

You are the connector, the mediator, the confidante, the sister, the partner, the friend, the dream-chaser, and so much more.

You are the heartbeat of the life you've built.

None of it exists without you, Mama. So, take care of yourself, meaningfully. Let self-care be more than a surface gesture. Let it truly replenish you. It's not just about feeling inspired, it's also about implementing practices into your life that restore your strength. Everything else can wait. Put on your own life jacket first before trying to keep everything and everyone else afloat; it's from this place of strength that you can best serve others.

Fill your soul cup with what fulfills you. Take deep breaths. Truly reflect on how far you've come and all the gratitude you feel for the life you've prayed for. I saw a bumper sticker recently that said *You are living at least one of the prayers you've prayed for.* It struck a deep chord in me.

What are you currently living with that is a prayer answered? Breathe it in. Soak it in. Steep in gratitude and love for it. For you.

(A PRAYER FOR TODAY)

My prayer in every moment is one of gratitude: thank you, thank you, thank you. May I continue to be the beacon of light, faith, love, hope, and courage that my baby, loved ones, and I need.

What are you celebrating right now?

I was leading a Mother's Circle today, and I asked what each mother was currently struggling with in their own journey. Most of the mothers shared a hardship, but one mother simply said she was in a really good place *at this moment*. It wasn't that she was finding motherhood easier than the rest, she was just in a particular period of celebration.

We often find it difficult to celebrate ourselves and our own growth.

Today, I want you to take a moment to celebrate all the things in your life that have you feeling excited and grateful. Even the smallest moments. It all counts.

Celebrate who you are. Celebrate your baby. Celebrate yourself as a mother.

Celebration is a beautiful frequency of love and gratitude woven together, which then only attracts more of the same. And hear this, Mama: You are not boastful or selfish for celebrating yourself. You are deserving of every ounce of joy you let yourself feel.

Soak in these times to sustain you through the moments that aren't as bright.

(A PRAYER FOR TODAY)

It's safe for me to celebrate the blessings in my life.

The energetics around you

Take a moment to pause and tune in. Whose energy are you carrying? Start with a deep breath in. Hold it briefly. Now exhale any tension you've been carrying (you may not even realize your body is holding on to something).

Do a full body scan. Notice your breath. Notice your heart. Notice where you feel dense, heavy, or unclear in your body. Is it your heart, belly, lower back, legs, shoulders, or head? Each area holds wisdom, connected to emotions that may need your attention:

Heart: relationships, betrayal, receiving love and support

Belly/Womb: boundary work, safety in your body, safety in finances, pressure and stress

Throat: communication, openness, truth-telling or holding back your truth

Lower Back: resentment, overperformance fatigue, safety, providership/ receivership

Legs: community, support, self-trust, foundational work

Shoulders: environmental/collective stress and tension, pressure of over-giving, over-functioning

Head: overthinking, living too much in the past or future

Whose energy are you carrying? Now, begin a practice of release. Repeat to yourself: "My energy is mine and stays with me. Your energy is yours and stays with you." Say it softly, firmly, and with intention.

Shake it off, dance it off, or bathe it out in an Epsom salt bath with some fresh eucalyptus leaves or oils. Release what was never yours to carry in the first place: other people's opinions, projections, and limitations, including your own Come back to your body, your breath, your remembrance of who you are here to be.

(A PRAYER FOR TODAY)

May I release everything that is not mine to carry and remember that I can call back my energy to me whenever I need it most. I rebuke all negative contacts and associations that siphon my energy. I stand strongly in my own energy and power.

Barefoot and balanced

What if I told you that one of the greatest anti-inflammatories and antiox-idants is free and right under your feet? Quite literally. Would you use it?

The practice of "grounding," or walking barefoot on the earth, is believed by many to be one of the most underrated health practices in our lifetime because it improves the function of almost every part of our body. Yet we rarely access it.

It sounds so simple, and it's tempting to shrug it off. But walking barefoot on the soil allows us to connect directly with the Earth's natural frequency, which is known scientifically as the Schumann Resonance and is lovingly referred to as the "Earth's heartbeat."

Grounding synchronizes our biological rhythms with the natural elec-tromagnetic current of nature, fostering a sense of rejuvenation. Feet to earth normalizes our circadian rhythm, inviting deeper, more restful sleep. Research has also shown that it increases blood flow to the face and body, helping with mobility and anti-aging. It's no coincidence that the Earth's heartbeat pulsates at 7.83 Hz, which is the same frequency as meditative alpha waves in the human brain. By absorbing the Earth's electrons through our feet, we help balance our body's own electrical state.

In this sacred communion with the earth, in addition to improving our overall well-being, we find balance, tranquility, and a profound sense of belonging. I don't know of any mother (including myself) who wouldn't benefit from a healthier, more-attuned vessel, less tension, deeper sleep, and a calmer alchemy of hormones. Basically, it's a full mind, body, and soul glow-up.

So, step outside today with your baby. Plant your bare feet (and perhaps their little toes too) upon the soil, aligning your whole being with the pulse of the planet.

(A PRAYER FOR TODAY)

God, thank you for the creation of this earth and the calming frequencies that pulse through it. May I embrace this nurturing energy as a way of connecting to you. Guide me to find moments of peace in nature and to draw strength from the world around me.

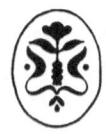

Sip of Self-Care:

Gardening with Intention

Take a moment to connect with the earth by planting something with your own hands. Whether it's a small flower, herb, or vegetable, let yourself be fully present as you dig into the soil. Feel its coolness and texture, grounding yourself in the moment.

With each movement, breathe deeply and connect to the Earth's heartbeat, allowing its calming energy to flow through you. This simple act of nurturing the earth also nurtures your spirit, helping you reconnect with balance and peace. Let the act of gardening ground you, bringing you back to a place of tranquility and renewal.

The same you, but different

No, you're not going "crazy," you're *still* navigating the ongoing waves of postpartum hormones. Postpartum isn't just the first few weeks or months after birth. It's a season of transformation that can stretch well into the first two years.

Be gentle with yourself, Mama.

I know some days the emotions will wash over like waves of a tsunami, without notice. Other days, you may feel calm, grounded, and content. Both are normal. It's okay to feel what you feel. And it's okay to seek support, whether it's a shoulder to lean on or professional help when it feels like the waves are pulling you under.

Your anxiety, obsessive thoughts, perfectionism, or sadness are part of your body's natural process of alchemizing the change, of recalibration. Postpartum is a journey, and healing takes time.

The key to finding your center again lies in surrounding yourself with the right support system, those who will hold space for your full humanity without judgment. Doing little sips of self-care that give you time and space to acclimatize with the transitions each phase of motherhood brings will fill you with more fuel to keep going. And seeking connections that feel safe yet expansive, where you feel seen and heard for who you are and who you are called to be, will continue to be the map to guide you in the right direction on your journey.

So today, take a deep breath, step outside, and feel the fresh air on your face. Look at your baby and marvel at how far you have come. And in case you haven't heard it today, you are doing an incredible job.

(A PRAYER FOR TODAY)

On days when I feel like the whirlwind of emotions never ends, guide me. Calm my heart. It's safe to feel what I feel. It's safe to seek support. It's safe to be witnessed in my full range of emotions.

Your environment is crucial to your well-being

As a new mom, your influence over your baby is powerful. The way you look at them, hold them, speak to them, and care for them all have an impact on their emotional and physical well-being. But have you ever thought about who you allow to influence you?

Motivational speaker Jim Rohn[12] famously said we're influenced by the five people we spend the most time with. However, it goes deeper than just your external surroundings. It's not just the people physically around you (your external environment), it's the voices you allow into your mind and heart (your internal environment) that profoundly shape your well-being.

Who do you listen to? What do you read? Whose social accounts do you choose to scroll through? Whose advice do you let steep into your consciousness? Are they living, parenting, and building their life in ways that align with you and who you desire to be?

These are important parts of your environment, the soil in which you are planted. In nature, proper soil composition provides essential minerals and elements, optimizes microbial activity, and ensures adequate aeration—the necessities not only for growth but also to form a protective barrier against disease and critters. The right environment gives the plant the best chance for overall resilience and vitality.

You are no different. Every so often, take time to evaluate your "soil." Who and what are you allowing into your life? Are they enriching your journey or pulling you away from your purpose?

(A PRAYER FOR TODAY)

God, surround me with people and influences that nourish my soul and my mind. Help me feel your guiding hand at every step of the way.

A note on memories

Do you know that it's our sensory inputs that imprint memories on our brain?

Think about a sweet memory from your childhood. For me, it's the feeling of warm towels fresh from the dryer. My mom would wrap us in them after long summer days in the pool. She was a teacher, so summers meant she was with us, savoring slow days together. My sisters and I would change into our pajamas in the middle of the day and take long naps. I can still smell the pizza from our local spot that we would grab on the way home.

What memory is nostalgic for you? Chances are it's woven with sensory details—the look, smell, taste, texture, or sound of something precious. Because that is how we remember. For me, warm towels and hot pizza will forever hold a special place in my heart.

You are in a season of planting seeds for new memories you are co-creating with your baby. I promise you, even though they may be too young to remember certain things right now, their subconscious is soaking it all in. And as they get older, they will start to consciously tuck those moments in the foundation of their being.

So, continue to invite your baby into the sensory world. Carry them to smell the flowers or encourage them to feel the ingredients of what you are cooking in their hands. Imprint the moments on both of your hearts.

(A PRAYER FOR TODAY)

Thank you, God, for the gift of presence and time with my baby. Thank you for the magic of memories with each other. May I continue to show up with love, gratitude, and peace, even on days when I'm not at my highest capacity. It's safe to be wholly me as I create new memories with my baby.

Whose story are you living today?

Is it yours? Is it one you've held on to from before your initiation into motherhood?

For me, stepping into motherhood meant confronting a story I didn't even realize I was clinging to. As an attorney, I had grown accustomed to viewing my time through the lens of "billable hours," measuring my worth by how much I produced. I tied my value to outcomes, deliverables, and the unrelenting grind of achievement. Even after stepping away from law-firm life into the nonprofit space, that mindset lingered. Motherhood, with all its messy, unquantifiable magic, forced me to reevaluate. Was I less valuable because I wasn't ticking off a checklist? Was my worth diminished because my productivity now looked like soothing a crying baby or folding laundry instead of drafting contracts?

The truth was, I needed to let go of that old story—the one that said my value came solely from output. I needed to embrace a new narrative, one that honored not just what I did but who I was becoming.

Whatever story is running the show for you, today is your chance to pause, reflect, and choose. Is it serving you? Does it honor the woman you are now? If not, it's time to let it go. You have the power to write a new narrative, one that calls you forward and honors your evolution.

Today is your day, Mama.

Revere the experiences that have gotten you here, then take a deep breath. Inhale and exhale. Step into the newness that awaits you in each moment.

Maybe it's even time to throw in a good plot twist.

(A PRAYER FOR TODAY)

Today, I choose to release the stories that hold me back or limit me in any way. Help me lean deeper into the narratives that reflect my evolution.

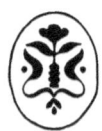

Sip of Self-Care:

Write Your Motherhood Word Bank: A Compass for Your Story

Take a moment to reflect on the essence of the motherhood story you want to create. What words capture the feelings, values, and energy you hope to embody? For me, words like "soft," "slow," and "adventurous" come to mind.

Write down at least twenty words that resonate with you, words that feel like the branches supporting the tree of your motherhood journey. Once you have your list, place it somewhere you'll see daily.

When you find yourself in a chapter that feels heavy or out of alignment, return to your word bank. Let it guide you back to the core of your story, helping you rewrite each new day with intention, grace, and clarity. These words are your anchor, your reminder of the beauty you're cultivating.

You can have faith or fear, not both

I know our mother hearts are tender and may lean toward worry, anxiousness, and fear of the unknown for our babies. We are hardwired to want to protect them in every way because they are extensions of our hearts and souls living outside our bodies. It is our sacred responsibility to nurture them, nourish them, protect them, guide them, love them, and empower them to thrive.

But here's the thing about fear: It's just information. It's not the enemy, it's courage announcing itself. Fear whispers of what matters most to us and invites us to step into bravery. You can choose faith or fear, but not both.

Faith is a bold declaration of trust, a steadying belief that everything is unfolding as it should. Fear, in contrast, is the absence of that trust, a tether to uncertainty. When we choose faith, we don't ignore the fear—we see it, name it, and then move forward courageously, carrying it with us as proof of what we hold dear.

Today, I pray that your faith is stronger than your fear.

I pray for trust within yourself, your heart, your strength, your baby's soul and purpose, and in the divine plan that binds you both. I pray that you continue to walk closely with God. I trust that everything will unfold for you and your baby as it's meant to.

(A PRAYER FOR TODAY)

I pray for deep trust within myself, my heart, my strength, my baby's soul, and their sacred mission on earth. May faith guide me, and may my fear be transformed into courage.

Fuel your body; nourish your spirit

As mothers, our bodies are tired. And sometimes, our spirits hover a few inches off the ground. Did you know that on average, moms lose three times more sleep than dads in the first year of parenthood? I came across that sobering statistic tonight while I was rocking my little one to sleep for the sixth time, and it's only 10 p.m.

In moments like these, I often ask myself: How can I rise in strength, both physically and spiritually?

What have you been doing to fuel your body these past few months? How have your energy levels been? Do you honor your physical capacity?

Let's remember that it's okay to feel different now. It's okay to need something new. See what micro-practices you can incorporate throughout the day—deep breaths while rocking your baby, a walk outside to feel the sunshine on your face, a quick shower to feel refreshed (this is my go-to).

Focus on nourishing your body, inside and out, through foods that comfort you, energize you, fuel you. Through movement that feels good. Through body treatments that restore you, cleanse you, and move the stagnant energy out.

How have you been nourishing your spirit? Nourish your soul and mind through mindful language, reflection, prayer, and meaningful connection. You are worthy of that care.

Whatever it is you most need, don't be afraid to give that to yourself in the ways that you can.

(A PRAYER FOR TODAY)

On days when I feel it all too strongly, guide me to my breath. May I continue to nourish my mind, body, spirit, and energy with all that brings me peace. May I see myself how you see me, God—whole, worthy, and radiant.

Water your relationships enough to thrive, not just survive

The lists will always be there . . .

The dishes will always need to be washed . . .

The laundry will always need to be folded . . .

The errands and chores will always need to be done . . .

Life can feel like an endless stream of tasks. And while those routines keep things running, don't let them drain the magic from your relationships with your partner, your baby, your friends and family, and most of all, yourself.

Before my partner and I got married, we learned about something called MIMs: Marriage Investment Minutes. It's a simple practice—a few intentional minutes set aside every week to truly connect on a deeper level. To pause the noise and tend to each other. MIMs taught us those relationships, like gardens, need daily care to flourish. It can be simple, and short. Just as long as it's something you come back to again and again. For us, it's going on a walk in the evening for fifteen to twenty minutes.

And it's not just in marriage; every relationship thrives when watered with attention, kindness, and a willingness to evolve. The time will pass anyway, but relationships wither without nourishment.

So, take a moment. Pause the lists, step away from the sink, let the laundry wait. Water your connections—whether that's a deep conversation, a shared laugh, or a quiet moment together. Only you know what your relationships need to not just survive, but truly thrive.

(A PRAYER FOR TODAY)

God, I am grateful for all the relationships in my life. May I remain present, attuned, and committed to nurturing them consistently, consciously.

Perhaps you are searching the branches for what only appears in the roots

Growth rarely happens exactly when or how we expect. Often, life unfolds in ways that feel delayed, misaligned, or completely out of our control.

But somehow, when we look back at the experience in the rearview mirror, it all makes sense. My partner and I went to the same college, were in the same year in school, and even had the same major, yet we didn't meet until years after we had both graduated and happened to be visiting a mutual friend in California on the same weekend. I thank God for that every day. This was God's timing. And the root of God's timing will always give us the more fruitful outcome.

So, release the timeline. Breathe in ease. Breathe out control.

Everything you desire and envision will happen for you, in time.

Release the preconceived timelines for your evolution, for your baby's milestones (even if there are guidelines to follow, remember they're just guidelines, not hard-and-fast rules). Trust the process, even when it's uncomfortable. You are stepping into a deeper initiation, growing stronger roots that will one day support an abundant bloom.

(A PRAYER FOR TODAY)

Teach me acceptance, surrender, and the art of letting go of all expectations. Not in my time, God, but yours.

Sip of Self-Care:

Embrace the Unfolding

Think back to a beautiful moment or milestone in your life—meeting your partner, discovering a deep friendship, or landing a dream opportunity. Recall its beginnings. What were you doing? What season of life were you in? Chances are, you weren't meticulously planning for it. Instead, life's unexpected twists, turns, and serendipitous timing led you there in ways you couldn't have predicted.

Let this reflection be a reminder that some of life's greatest gifts come not from forcing outcomes, but from releasing the timeline and trusting the flow. When you loosen your grip on what "should" happen and when, you create space for God to surprise you in ways far beyond what you could imagine. Lean into the unfolding. Life's magic often blooms in the spaces where we let go.

Nourish new roots

An interesting fact about roots is that their growth happens almost exclusively underground, in the dark, out of sight from the external world. Yet this process is arguably the most important part for the health of the plant. These roots determine the nourishment that the plant will receive, the location on which it will rest, and therefore, the site for its offspring for generations to come.

You are in a season of rooting in your motherhood. Let new roots take place. Let new roots anchor you into your faith, your self-confidence, your love and leadership as a mother and woman.

Anchor new roots in your relationship with yourself, your body, your baby, your family, your friends, and your partner. This growth may also be happening beneath the surface, but tending to these tentacles is nourishment for the foundation of your mothering journey and future environment.

Let new roots ground you; trust that this is a necessary part of your story.

(A PRAYER FOR TODAY)

May the roots I plant deepen and grow into a beautiful bloom that is motherhood.

Don't limit yourself

I know this might sound strange at first, especially when you've been told your whole life that you need to pick one thing to do or be really good at in order to be successful, but don't put yourself in a box.

I have always struggled with this concept, and the debate in my head of "who I am" got even louder and more conflicted once I became a mother. The world tells us that in order to do something well, we have to focus on that one thing. But we are women with many interests and skill sets. The feminine energy pulsating through our being cannot be confined to a box or a label. Labels are limiting—and you, my dear, are *limitless*.

So, let me remind you: You get to be it all—the multi-passionate, multifaceted human being you were born to be. You don't have to choose between either/ or, or ever give yourself an ultimatum (unless you need to in order to reach a decision that is in your highest attunement).

As a mother, you get to embody any of or all the archetypes you want—the mother, the woman, the artist, the lover and partner, the entrepreneur, the career woman, the nurturer, the best friend, the chef, the adventurer.

And who doesn't love choices?

(A PRAYER FOR TODAY)

God, may I remember that you created me as a human being with many layers, unique interests, and talents. Guide me to show up unapologetically and shine my light boldly and brightly.

Your rebirth is unfurling

In the tender embrace of spring, nature whispers of rebirth all around us. Buds unfurl like secrets, and the earth awakens in a symphony of new life. Here you stand, Mama, nearly nine months into motherhood.

How are you feeling? What is awakening within you?

I know despite how much we plan for something, change is never easy. However, what helps us integrate it deeply and with ease is *allowing* ourselves to evolve into the new lifestyle we are being called to live.

Does your life support this rebirth? How does it feel now versus when you were first initiated into motherhood? What are some things that have worked really well for you? What are some edges of growth you'd love to continue leaning deeper into? What are some things that no longer work that you are now called to release?

Journal this out, record it, or connect with a trusted friend about it. If you have a partner, do a check-in.

I promise you, this evolution is happening for you and for your baby. Each budding flower in your life is a testament to the ever-turning wheel of birth, death, and renewal.

(A PRAYER FOR TODAY)

God, help me create a supportive environment for my new life, my evolved self, that is preparing to bloom in motherhood.

Your life is not a zero-sum game

Tonight, I hosted a meditation event for mothers in Chicago. It was a success by many standards, and it felt good to be heard and seen and to hold space for these incredible women . . . until I got home and felt the wave of guilt wash over me. I had missed bedtime with my son. In moments like this, I find myself wondering: When I pour into my personal aspirations, am I falling short as a mother? Are my dreams at odds with my mothering journey? What is this elusive balance I'm searching for?

My fear is that I will always be longing for the other side: In a stretch of time with my baby, will I wish I had more time for myself? In taking time for myself, will I long to be back with my baby? And so it goes, the never-ending loop of mom guilt—a cycle that makes it feel like life is a zero-sum game, where one area must lose for the other to gain. But that's not how life works. *It is not a zero-sum game.*

Your life is not a winner-takes-all competition. You can thrive in both your passions and your mothering journey. Whether it's taking the night to yourself or spending time with your child, you "win" either way because in each scenario you are expanding in some way.

What is the right balance between your passions and your purpose in mothering? Only you know, but remember that it doesn't have to be all or nothing.

(A PRAYER FOR TODAY)

In those moments when I am quick to be hard on myself, may I remember that no one loves my child more than I do, and I have everything I need within me. Thank you, God, for entrusting me in this role as the mother to my sweet child.

Sip of Self-Care:

Affirmations for Embracing Duality

When mom guilt creeps in, remind yourself of this truth: life is not a zero-sum game, and two things can be true at once. Repeat these words to yourself:

- "I will honor the duality of motherhood and selfhood. By filling my own cup, I create more love, energy, and presence to pour into my family."

Let this affirmation ground you in the understanding that your well-being and dreams don't diminish your motherhood, they enrich it. You are creating a life where both you and your baby can thrive.

Clarity is sometimes found in movement rather than stillness

I have realized since becoming a mother how often my inner perfectionism takes the wheel. And when she's driving, we don't get very far. We can't, as we are constantly evaluating and reevaluating, assessing and reassessing, mapping it out and then looking for alternative routes.

There are so many directions I envision for my life's work, my passions, and my mothering. And you may be feeling this too. So where do you start?

The answer: Anywhere.

Because what's in motion continues to compound and stays in motion. So, today's reminder is to not give up on the things that matter to you or spend energy trying to rush or chase your dreams on everyone else's timelines.

Set your intentions, then try them on with small, simple actions (even if it is one tiny thing a day). Choose quality over quantity. Do the things that matter to you versus those that the world tells you need to be done. We often think that clarity requires stillness, but we can gain so much insight from just starting. From dipping our toes in the water and watching the ripples. From there, you can always sidestep, pivot, or change course entirely.

Focus on turning the wheels of the healing, the growth, and the evolution and expansion you are being led to in each moment, no matter how slow it may appear from the outside looking in. What matters most is taking the first step, even if imperfect.

Choose to keep going. Choose to show up for yourself and your baby in ways that you are able, one day at a time.

(A PRAYER FOR TODAY)

May I have the courage to keep showing up. May I put in motion those things that matter most to me.

Follow your soul fire

You may feel that soul nudge from time to time in this season.

Where your whole body ignites with the desire to do something different. Maybe it's to take a power pause and fully be enveloped in motherhood. Perhaps it's an itch to begin a new creative or business venture, to explore a new hobby, or to pursue a new direction career-wise. Now that motherhood has initiated you into an elevated frequency, you may feel discernment rising within you.

Wherever you find yourself, Mama, honor that soul fire. It's healing for you and your baby. It is helping you break generational anchors and chart a brand-new adventure for yourself. We often dim or extinguish our soul fire because we subscribe to the traditional adages of parenthood and mother-hood, either from how we've grown up or what we've witnessed within the women in our family and group of friends.

I'm here to tell you, you don't have to lose yourself or your soul in the whirlpool of motherhood. A child is a great motivation to inhabit a brighter existence. Let motherhood fuel you forward, however that looks for you. Maybe that means finally slowing down or simplifying your life.

I have dear friends who had businesses but put them on pause because their soul longed to be with their child (that took courage). I have others (myself included) who love motherhood but also felt called, for any number of reasons, to continue pursuing passions outside of mothering in a way that works for them. Everything is okay as long as you tend to *your* soul's fire and no one else's.

(A PRAYER FOR TODAY)

God, teach me to hear your voice. Reignite my inner fire and help me shine my light and speak my truth. Give me the courage to pursue the calling you've placed in my heart. Let motherhood be my stronghold and anchor that propels me forward.

Worrying is a waste of imagination

It was my first week at a law firm after finishing school. I was the youngest (and most inexperienced) attorney on staff, and I could barely keep my breakfast down as I sat in my new office and stared at the contract I had been asked to review.

Then, as if summoned by my anxiety, one of the named partners appeared in my doorway. He was in his seventies, a legend in the field. "You look worried," he observed, leaning casually against the doorframe.

I managed a small chuckle and admitted, "This is all very new."

What he said next has stuck with me for the past fifteen years: "Don't be. Worrying is a waste of the imagination. You'll need your mind for other things."

It's the best advice I've ever received. Rationally, we know deep down anxiety serves no real purpose. But let's be honest, it's easier said than done. Especially as mothers. The future beckons with all our plans and possibilities, tempting us to get lost in its hypothetical "what-ifs." Meanwhile, the past tugs at us with its lessons and regrets, drawing us into a spiral of "what could have been." I've lived in both places. Yet we cannot change the past, only remember it and sit with the emotions that surface.

As for the future? We can't control that either. The present moment is where life happens, Mama. It's where you'll find joy, connection, and the clarity you seek.

So today, when you notice your thoughts drifting—whether to a future that feels overwhelming or to past wounds that no longer serve you—pause. Take a few deep breaths. There is no need to be anxious about what is yet to come.

It's a waste of your precious brain power, your time, and most importantly, *your imagination.*

(A PRAYER FOR TODAY)

Quell my anxious spirit, and give me peace of mind, body, and soul. I trust that what is best for me and my family will not pass us by. It will unfold as it's meant to be.

A catalyst for clarity

You are multidimensional.

So, your purpose is multidimensional too, Mama. It's safe to claim it, boldly and out loud.

Motherhood can be your greatest expander and initiation, if you allow it to be. Feel the bigness of the power that you wield as a creator. Stand rooted in it, unapologetically.

When you step into matrescence, it can feel like the waters of your soul are stirred, kicking up the sand and making everything seem murky. Yet as the sand settles, clarity begins to emerge. Motherhood can become a profound catalyst for that clarity. Suddenly your time, energy, and presence—the most finite of resources—are illuminated, their value heightened. This newfound awareness sharpens your ability to discern what truly deserves your attention. So, what are those multidimensional dreams and ventures your soul is being called toward either now or in the future?

Write them out. Think about them, visualize them, pray over them. Allow them to unfold in their own divine timing. And please remember that having other dreams alongside motherhood does not make you less of a mother. The journey of your life is long, with many seasons to embrace. If this season calls you to focus solely on motherhood, let yourself savor it fully. If it calls you to pursue something beyond, honor that too. You hold the wisdom to know what is best for you and your family.

You are meant for everything your heart desires and more.

(A PRAYER FOR TODAY)

God, remind me of my strength and clear the path for any dreams that are in my heart to unfold in your timing.

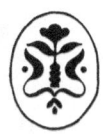

Sip of Self-Care:

Exploring Your Many Layers

Labels can be both empowering and limiting, but they don't have to define your entire story. Instead, think of them as windows into the many roles, passions, and possibilities that make up who you are.

Today, take a moment to reflect on your multifaceted self. Make a list of all the things that spark your curiosity, the hobbies you've dabbled in, and the dreams you long to explore. Include the roles you hold—mother, partner, friend, creator, etc., including the parts of you that often go unnoticed.

Let this list remind you that you are not one thing but a beautifully layered being with endless potential. This exercise isn't about pinning yourself down, it's about expanding your sense of who you are and who you're becoming.

Eventually, all waves settle

Life isn't always smooth sailing, but hopefully you're starting to realize that you are resilient and strong for navigating the waves of motherhood the way you do. For weaving your life together the way that you do.

For nurturing your baby the way you do. For choosing *you* and your evolution in ways that feel nourishing to you. For loving yourself and your family the way you do. For weathering the hard days and the in-between moments.

Today, take a moment to celebrate you, Mama. You've made it this far. Remember that all waves eventually settle. You are finding your rhythm, and you're doing a really beautiful job.

(A PRAYER FOR TODAY)

Thank you, God, for making me resilient. Show me that my strength lies in both my resilience and my softness.

Self-care as a declaration

Too often I hear from mothers about how guilty they feel for taking time for themselves. I've felt that too, which is one of the reasons that I've peppered this book with self-care tips. Even though we know that taking care of ourselves is important for both our emotional and physical well-being, we still feel guilty about taking "me" time. As new moms, we want to pour everything we have into our babies. But what happens when we're drained with nothing left to give?

It took me a while to realize that a mother who feels supported and emotionally cared for can nurture a more positive relationship with her child. Taking care of myself isn't selfish, it's essential. My well-being trickles out to my family, and I am the anchor of my baby's emotional well-being.

But self-care is deeply personal. Nobody else is living *your* motherhood.

Only you know what you most need, so today I invite you to give yourself whatever that is as part of your self-care routine. It could be taking some quiet time in the bath or ordering takeout while you rest with the baby instead of cooking. Or maybe it's hiring a cleaning service once a month. Perhaps you want to adjust your space to suit this new initiation and evolution of motherhood. Whatever it is, know you are worthy of it all.

Remember that these practices are making you stronger, and your strength is what carries your family.

So, make your declaration, and tend to yourself too, Mama.

(A PRAYER FOR TODAY)

Guide me to honor my soul and to nurture the light within in ways that feel aligned. May I remember that caring for myself is an act of devotion.

Motherhood is a creative playground

There is nothing like motherhood to teach you how to adapt at a moment's notice, how to improvise and make strawberry jam out of strawberries, and how to play—truly let go and *play* in each moment—even when life feels like a chaotic storm. Like the time I lost my wallet in the middle of a busy day, with my baby in tow. For a moment, panic surged through me. But then I looked at my son, his wide eyes absorbing my every reaction, and I knew that this was a moment to practice what I preach.

Babies are incredibly perceptive. They feel our energy, attune to our nervous system, and sense how calm or frazzled we really are beneath the surface. No matter what we say to our babies, they can decipher the feelings behind the words. Adults can fool other adults, but we can't fool our babies.

So as I stood there, wallet nowhere to be found, I took a deep breath and imagined the story I wanted my son to internalize. Not one of stress or spiraling frustration, but one of resilience and adaptability. I decided to turn it into a game: searching every pocket, retracing steps, making a scavenger hunt out of the moment. My son giggled at the exaggerated "uh-ohs" and cheered when I finally found the wallet wedged between his diaper bag straps. What could have been a meltdown transformed into a memory.

Motherhood has this wild way of stretching you. It's a leadership role like no other, where your creative freedom and ability to stay grounded have lasting ripple effects. These everyday moments—the messy, unexpected ones—are the building blocks that shape your baby's memory bank. They store not just what we do but how we feel while we do it.

What if we approached the next chaotic moment with a sense of play? What if, instead of stress, we zoomed out, calmed our hearts, and made the best of what's in front of us?

Motherhood is a playground that invites you to innovate. Allow yourself to have fun with it while your little one is watching you shine.

(A PRAYER FOR TODAY)

May I see life's hurdles as opportunities to get creative in my solutions as I model to my baby how to weave in and through situations, conflicts, and emotions.

There is nothing stronger than a mother

Whatever it is you put your mind and soul to, embrace it like a mother.

Love like a mother.

Fight fiercely and fairly like a mother.

Advocate relentlessly like a mother.

Stand tall and proud in your strength like a mother.

Laugh like a mother.

Cry like a mother.

Open your heart like a mother.

Revere who you are like a mother.

Soften and surrender like a mother.

Pursue your dreams like a mother.

Walk in your fullest power like a mother.

Which one of these attitudes do you need to embody the most today? Say it out loud. Write it on your mirror or a sticky note and put it wherever you need to see it.

(A PRAYER FOR TODAY)

God, help me remember that the title of Mother is one that you bestowed on me. Help me walk in this capacity with confidence and a relentless love.

Sip of Self-Care:

Aligning Heart and Mind: A Self-Love Practice

Find a quiet moment to center yourself. Place one hand gently on your forehead and the other on your heart. Close your eyes and take a deep, grounding breath. As you do, invite your heart to lead, asking your mind to step back and support its wisdom. Visualize your head and heart merging, working together as a single, harmonious unit—connected, intuitive, and aligned.

Breathe deeply here for twenty cycles, allowing this union to settle into your being. As you breathe, curl your lips into a soft smile, feeling the kindness and warmth of that expression radiating through your face. Let that gentle, joyous energy shine inward, illuminating every corner of your being.

This is your light, your love, reflecting back upon yourself. Stay here as long as you like, basking in the harmony of head and heart working as one.

You are limitless

I'll never forget the day I realized how much my energy shaped my little one's world. My son was almost nine months old, a bundle of curiosity and giggles, watching me with those wide, trusting eyes. It had been one of those mornings with barely any sleep and a long list of things to do. I felt so small, buried under the weight of it all. But then I looked at him and his face lit up just because I was there. And I thought: *What if I show him what it means to choose joy, even on the tough days?*

So, I wrapped him in my arms, left the chaos behind, and stepped outside. The sky was gray and heavy, and as if on cue, the rain began to fall. Instead of running back inside, we stayed. I twirled in the rain, holding him close, his little body bouncing with each spin. He laughed so hard it turned into hiccups, and I couldn't stop laughing with him.

That moment cracked something open in me. Motherhood isn't about shrinking under the weight, it's about letting it stretch us into something bigger.

Mama, you are not here to play small. When you live boldly and unapologetically, you show your baby—your adorable little sponge of a human—that life is to be *lived*.

Carry your baby out into the world. Sit in the grass, feel the mud between your fingers, let the rain soak your hair. Buy yourself flowers for no reason; show your child what it means to embrace life fully.

(A PRAYER FOR TODAY)

Thank you, God, for making me a powerhouse and for sending me the wind of life to make my inner flame burn bright. You have created me for so much goodness; allow me see it and find my stride.

Trust the seeds you are planting

Nine months—this is a huge milestone, Mama! I hope you are celebrating yourself today.

Your motherhood is much like a garden. There are seeds that you plant now, then water and nurture, that will yield a beautiful bloom as time goes on. You have spent nine months planting, nurturing, protecting, and watering the seeds of your relationship with yourself and with your tiny human.

Nine months experiencing milestones together, journeying together, learning each other's energetic cadences and languages, and allowing your personalities to evolve and develop together.

Nine months of you stepping into the most powerful initiation as a woman.

Nine months of you and your body contracting, expanding—metaphorically and literally—physically, hormonally, mentally, and emotionally.

Nine months of you forging your own path of motherhood.

I am so proud of you! I know the journey hasn't always been easy. But look how far you've come.

So here's to you; here's to the beautiful baby you're raising; here's to the family you're growing and the chosen family you're welcoming into your life.

(A PRAYER FOR TODAY)

Thank you for these first nine months of my journey as a mother. Thank you for helping me birth my baby and bring them earthside. Thank you for the rebirth of my soul as a mother. Thank you, thank you, thank you.

(Summer)

THE MOTHER'S BLOOM

THE FOURTH QUARTER:

AWAKENING, EXPANSION, INTEGRATION

"The brightest flowers can only bloom after the rain."

*Scan for meditations to guide you
through this season*

Summer: The Mother's Bloom
AWAKENING . EXPANSION . INTEGRATION

Here we are together in the final season of our Mother Year, Summer. This is a season of integration, meaning to "blend into a functioning or unified whole." How does reading that definition land in your heart? Do you feel like the parts of yourself are being woven back together, perhaps in an even more healed and unified way than before becoming a mother? Do you now feel more in sync with how you flow daily with your baby than those first few months? You have been through so much in your Mother Year, and in this season, we celebrate every decision, cry, laugh, late night, early morning, hard day, and grateful moment that this year has brought into your life.

You have lived and learned, released parts of yourself, and cultivated new ones. My hope is that you now feel in closer alignment to your worth, power, and ability to not only mother but also to show up as the strong, powerful woman you are and always have been.

In our Summer season, we fan the flame from the embers you've tended to all these months. And it is this fire within that will keep you warm in the many seasons of motherhood ahead, for Summer is simultaneously the last season in your Mother Year as well as the beginning of the next chapter ahead following your baby's first birthday. You see, we are constantly growing and beginning again. Like a flower that is planted, then blooms, withers, and returns to the soil, we, too, remain in a cyclical pattern. In motherhood, how you do the work *is the work*. There is no end "goal" to reach; rather, it's moment to moment—it's the ebb and flow of doing the best we can with the information in front of us. We will rewrite our story over and over again. We will bloom many times along the way. We often think of the "bloom" as the pinnacle, the climax of the story, but it's not—it's simply another point along the way with its own attributes. Still, it is full but fleeting.

So, in this Summer season, I offer these words to hold and guide you:

- Whatever makes you feel the sun from the inside out, chase that.
- Let love grow new roots in your heart.

- The joy of being human is not knowing what you will discover next.
- Your deep reservoir of ability and love has no end.
- Nurture a kind inner voice.
- Show yourself the same mothering energy that you do your baby.
- Fill your own cup so full that you can give and still be overflowing.
- You are a multifaceted human being; it's okay to tend to all parts of yourself.
- Flowers need time to bloom, and so do you.

You've got this, Mama.

Let motherhood rearrange you

Motherhood is here to transform you, if you allow it. Allow it to soften any hard edges of your soul and replace them with boundaries you didn't realize you needed. Allow it to humble you in the valleys right before introducing you to the highest mountain peaks of your life—peaks you will one day look back at in awe, marveling at the strength it took to scale them.

Motherhood is a sacred transformation, a process that breaks you open only to fill you with more love, wisdom, and strength than you ever thought possible. If you don't open your eyes, you may miss just how different you have become.

Be with it, sit with it, and breathe it in; feel it reverberate to your core. Let it rearrange you in the way that it was always meant to, even if that means you sometimes don't recognize the person staring back at you in the mirror.

You are blooming, Mama, so let it be *big*.

(A PRAYER FOR TODAY)

God, you are welcome here in my heart, and I trust you to do your work within me, through me, and through the miracle of life you have placed in my care. I am open to letting it transform me according to your plan.

Find your reason for being

Sometimes when I'm immersed in the whirlwind of sleepless nights, feedings, transitions, and the seemingly ceaseless demands of nurturing my baby, questions about my purpose swirl in my mind.

This longing for answers led me to *ikigai*, a Japanese philosophy that means "a reason for being." It's about finding purpose at the intersection of what you love, what you're good at, what the world needs, and what can support you financially. *Ikigai* teaches that meaning is found in small, daily actions that bring joy and fulfillment.

I began by reflecting on what lights up my heart, even when I'm exhausted. I thought about my strengths and how they could provide value to others. Finally, I contemplated what the world needs in this moment, realizing that raising a compassionate child is one of the most meaningful contributions I could make. This process helped me uncover my own *ikigai*—a blend of motherhood and my passions, which brought clarity to my days, turning ordinary routines into purposeful actions.

I am learning to balance love, purpose, and personal growth, weaving them into a life that feels truly meaningful.

Motherhood became not just a role but a journey toward discovering who I am and what truly matters. It's not about whether you stay home or work outside the house, it's about zooming out to reflect on your life as a whole, like a bird scanning the treetops for the path ahead. In the end, *ikigai* isn't a destination but a continuous journey of growth and self-discovery. It reminds us to embrace both the joys and challenges of motherhood while also nurturing the other aspects of our identity, in whatever form that may take.

(A PRAYER FOR TODAY)

God, fill my heart with clarity and joy as I uncover the profound meaning in my life. Let my purpose unfold naturally, like a blossom revealing its petals in the light of your love.

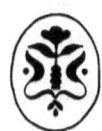

Sip of Self-Care:

Create your own *ikigai* map. Draw four overlapping circles and label them as such: "What I Love," "What I'm Good At," "What the World Needs Now," and "What Can Sustain Me?" Fill each circle with ideas, then look at the center where they overlap. This is your *ikigai*—a guide to living with purpose. Revisit and adjust it as your insights evolve.

Embrace your childlike spirit

Summer is a time of flourishing, a season that invites joy and play into our lives. As you navigate this chapter of your Mother Year, you may be discovering that you're not only finding your footing but also beginning to find your stride. The early months of motherhood, often filled with uncertainty, might now feel like a blur in the rearview mirror.

I think back to a quiet summer afternoon not long ago when I laid my baby down on a blanket under the shade of a tree in the park. He stared up at the swaying leaves, completely captivated. I found myself captivated too—not just by the leaves, but by the wonder in his eyes, the simplicity of his awe. In that moment, I realized how much beauty is in the small things I so often overlook. In this vibrant season, take a moment to stop and truly smell the roses as they bloom around you. It's easy to let the days slip by in a flurry of activity, ticking off milestones and accomplishments as if they are mere checkboxes rather than small miracles unfolding before your eyes.

Slow down and immerse yourself in the beauty and bounty that this season has to offer, knowing that all will come in divine timing. Allow yourself to enjoy these precious moments—the laughter, the quiet snuggles, the everyday victories. Every step you take is a part of a larger, divine rhythm that guides you and your child. Your journey, rich with its own experiences and joys, is a celebration of the love and growth that define this remarkable season of your life.

(A PRAYER FOR TODAY)

God, may I recognize feelings of ease and joy as they are happening.

Mothering outside the lines

I have spent most of my life doing what is expected of me, from taking my role as the eldest sibling seriously to pursuing law school, from getting married to moving through a series of coveted jobs as an attorney. At one point, I was living the quintessential life: a nice condo in Chicago, a goldendoodle named Remi, and all the milestones of a picture-perfect adulthood. And while there is nothing wrong with these classically defined milestones of adulthood, I can see now that, in some ways, they were guided by the quiet longing for external validation and collective belonging.

But becoming a mother awakened something fierce and steadfast within me—a deep, undeniable knowing that my mothering journey is uniquely mine. The experts don't know my child, nor do the authors of books. My mothering doesn't fit squarely into any prescribed belief system or parenting framework, and that's exactly how it should be. Instead, I am taking pieces that inspire me and making the mosaic of my motherhood journey for *us*.

It takes courage to step off the well-trodden path, to resist the urge to compare your child—or yourself—to a standard rooted in the so-called average. After all, none of us hope our children will be merely average. We don't want their lives to blend in, we want their unique light to shine. So why, then, would we measure them by a benchmark that disregards their individuality? What if our willingness to defy those norms, to trust our intuition, is the very sign that we're on the right path?

(A PRAYER FOR TODAY)

God, I am weary of following the molds that the world tries to fit me in. Lead me to trust you instead; let me rebel against a world that doesn't know me or my child like you do.

The sacred keeper

You are the weaver of dreams and souls, Mama, spinning the threads of love and hope with every touch.

You are the keeper of secrets, a best friend and confidante.

You are the sacred wellspring that gives life to your family, to your legacy, to your lineage.

You are the author of your life, your story, and the storyline that will shape your baby's world.

You are the compass they will look to for guidance.

You are the rock on which they will stand.

May you always be rooted in truth, in love, in your soul essence—one with God.

You are the sacred keeper—not only of your child's heart, their light, and their soul, but also of your own. As you nurture and protect their unique spark, you are called to honor your own essence, to tend to the sacred fire within you. You hold the bridge between who they are now and who they are becoming, while also tending to the path of your own unfolding, with infinite tenderness and grace. If you embrace it, motherhood will become the season that prunes and blooms you, refining you into your fullest, most beautiful self.

(A PRAYER FOR TODAY)

God, attune me daily to the needs of my soul and the needs of my child's soul. May I see them as they are, as you created them to be, not as I wish for them to be.

God lives all around us and within us

Some people think of God as someone sitting high in the sky on a throne. Instead, what if we believe he is woven within all natural things, including us. We are part of nature too.

What if he is in the trees above us and in the grass below our feet? What if he lives under our ribs within our heart space?

I love the idea that God inhabits all spaces and faces because it encourages us to see it all—our bodies, our baby, the earth—as sacred. And when we see them as sacred, we interact with them differently, caring for them with kindness, and expecting to feel the spirit in their presence.

So, what if you walked outside your door right now and could hear messages and answers to your prayers in the wind? In your own breath? Would you listen a little more carefully and walk more slowly around this earth?

(A PRAYER FOR TODAY)

God, I open myself up to you and your guidance. Thank you for the beauty that surrounds me and the sacredness with which you created all living things. Let me be a vessel for your messages and an example of how a full, colorful life looks.

Sip of Self-Care:

A Tiny Bouquet for You

Motherhood is a constant act of arranging—meals, naps, tiny clothes in drawers. Let yourself arrange something just for the beauty of it.

The next time you step outside, gather a few small blooms, a sprig of greenery, even wildflowers from the cracks in the sidewalk. Place them in a jar, a mug, or whatever you have nearby. Let the act be simple, instinctual—no need for perfection.

As you place each stem, imagine arranging a bit of beauty back into your own day. A reminder that, like these flowers, you are growing, unfolding, and worthy of sacred care.

You are all they need

My son was having a hard time falling asleep last night. He was calm in his crib, until he wasn't, then he began to cry. I walked into the room, and his cry lowered. I picked him up, and he almost immediately sank his heavy head to my chest. I sat down in the rocking chair and began singing to him. Within five minutes, he was completely asleep.

As I sat there rocking, it dawned on me how amazing it is that my voice soothes him, my touch puts him at ease, my presence makes him feel safe enough to rest, truly rest, without inhibition.

In my arms, his whole body recognizes my heart, my soul, and my smell. My very being is all he needs. I invite you today to remember that you are the only mother in the world perfectly attuned to your baby. What a miraculous thought that one person can have that level of calming effect on another, and you get to be that person for your child.

(A PRAYER FOR TODAY)

God, thank you for making me the vessel your love flows through to my baby. May I reflect on the comfort and ease you give to us.

Laughter is medicine

There are going to be lots of times you get it right, Mama. You know what I mean: those moments when you are ultra-prepared and have everything you need packed perfectly in the diaper bag. But there will also be times when you don't, and it might be messy. You need to find the humor in it. Laughter really is the best medicine; it's the antidote to self-criticism, a reminder that the little mishaps have no bearing on our worth as a mother. What makes us a good mother is our ability to be human, to make mistakes and learn from them, to grow, evolve, and change, and to be flexible for the experiences we don't see coming.

One time I forgot a change of clothes for my baby, so after an unexpected blowout, I had to use my scarf to make a Peter Pan outfit for him for the remainder of dinner. Was it chaos? Absolutely. But now it makes for a great story, and when I reflect on it, I still giggle.

So, take the medicine now, Mama. Laugh. It's good for the soul.

(A PRAYER FOR TODAY)

God, let me see the little messes as blessings I can infuse levity into as I make my way through this motherhood journey. May I cloak myself with the same medicine of kindness and grace that I offer my child.

Your mind and your body may not always be in the same place

It's okay to miss your baby while you're out for an evening with your partner, family, or friends. Your very first night out for more than an hour in what seems like months? Or maybe it's not new but an extension of the initial twenty-minute coffee dates and chats. Yet you find yourself missing your baby while you're away from them, even though you've been needing and desiring this time for a while. Mama, it's completely normal.

Your baby is safe and secure, wrapped in the warmth of familiar arms and soothed by voices they will come to know. Each time you step away, you're not just taking a break for yourself, you're also giving your baby the chance to bond with others who adore them. It's a dance of independence and connection, a rhythm that you and your little one will grow into together.

In this space of longing and loving, you're teaching your baby that while you may not always be physically present, your love never wavers. Every hug, every kiss, every whispered word of affection you give before you leave lingers in their heart. And when you return, the joy of reunion, the soft, sweet smiles, and the excited giggles strengthen your bond even further.

So, embrace the time you have for yourself. Let it refresh you, fill your cup, and remind you of the multifaceted woman you are. This balance, though delicate, is the foundation of a beautiful, resilient motherhood. You're not just stepping out, you're stepping *into* your full self, showing your baby that love can stretch across moments and miles, while always finding its way back home.

(A PRAYER FOR TODAY)

I am grateful for my village for loving my baby and wrapping them in their nurturing care and for supporting me and my family as we grow together. Thank you for the gentle hands that hold my child when I am away, for the kind words that soothe and comfort, and for the shared laughter that brightens our days. Bless these dear souls who stand by my side.

Your mental and energetic "diet" matters

Your mental and energetic "diet" matters more than you might realize.

When we hear the word "diet," our mind instantly thinks of food. But our diet is much more than that—it's simply what we consume regularly. It's the total intake of everything we ingest on a physical, emotional, and spiritual level in a given day. It is the shows we watch, the podcasts we listen to, the friends we converse with, the social media accounts we follow.

Be mindful of what you put in and around your mind and body because it has a profound effect on the way you feel about yourself and your life. It's all input and can make a difference in the way that you are showing up for yourself and for your baby (your output).

Your "diet" doesn't just affect you, it sets the tone for your whole family. So, choose wisely. Fill your life with joy, inspiration, and nourishment that uplifts and truly *sustains* you. Let it ground and energize you, rather than leaving you feeling drained or depleted.

(A PRAYER FOR TODAY)

May I have the power to see clearly when something is for me or against me, and may I have the courage to rid my life of anything that brings me out of alignment with my worthiness or my relationship with you, God.

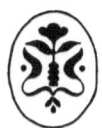

Sip of Self-Care:

Today, take a mindful pause to assess your mental and energetic "diet." Choose one habit—be it a TV show, a social media
account, or a recurring conversation—that doesn't uplift you.
Gently let it go and replace it with something that brings joy
and nourishment to your spirit.

Our babies understand the assignment

Society has tried to define what a "good" baby looks like: one that cries infrequently, sleeps on demand, and eats at regular intervals.

Hmm, that doesn't sound like a baby to me, it sounds like a robot. And it doesn't exist. (Nor would I want it to. I love my human baby just fine, thank you.)

The quicker we reset our expectations and realize that we gave birth to a warm-blooded human being whose needs, wants, and habits change daily, just as our own do, the more we can enjoy this period. We can be curious observers rather than trying to crack an impossible code to yield a "good baby."

The truth is that crying is communicating. We want our babies to speak. Our babies are meant to communicate their needs to us in the only way they can.

The truth is that they are meant to spit out food they don't recognize the textures of yet. They are learning their palate. They are supposed to throw food on the floor. They are learning what gravity is and how their hands and mouth work together.

They are meant to see us as a safe space to test boundaries so they can grow with confidence. They know they can take that step because we will catch them. They scream and pout because they know we will love them despite of it, and they are learning the full range of emotions available to them.

As strange as it may sound, most of the hard parts of motherhood really involve us allowing our children to *do their job.* Because their job is to just simply learn how to be a human being, having a somatic (bodily) experience in this world.

Let this reframe ease your mind. You are doing your job, Mama, and your baby is doing theirs.

(A PRAYER FOR TODAY)

God, thank you for the creative ways you have designed all babies, including mine, to grow and develop. Help me be a safe place for them to flourish. May I have the wisdom to guide my child on their own path.

Be realistic; plan for a miracle

My father was taken to the hospital at this time in my motherhood journey. It was in the height of the COVID pandemic, and he was quickly placed on a ventilator because he was having such a difficult time breathing. No one was allowed in to see him because of the hospital protocols at the time, and speaking on the phone was hard for him because of his fatigued airways. At one point, the doctor said that the following twenty-four hours would be critical as he would either take a turn for the worse, which could be fatal, or start to heal and make a full recovery. Hearing these words was bone-chilling. I sobbed on the phone with my father as he told me not to worry in a low, raspy voice.

It was terrifying, and we all felt so helpless. My mom, sisters, brother, and I scheduled a group call to pray for my father, asking for a miracle.

As I got off the phone, I held my son in my arms, my tears dripping down my face onto his blanket. It then dawned on me—I am holding a miracle in my arms.

God is so powerful. He created the very idea of life, and he can turn the smallest, tiniest egg into a human being. There is nothing he can't do. I prayed again, this time with a little more hope in my heart.

My father made a full recovery and was released from the hospital three days later. It would be hard, even impossible I would argue, to be a mother and not believe in miracles.

You have held it in your hands, felt it in your body.

Look around you, Mama, and expect miracles at every turn.

(A PRAYER FOR TODAY)

God, give me the courage to believe in miracles, the patience to await their arrival, and the gratitude to recognize them when they unfold. With trust in your divine plan, I eagerly anticipate the miracles that lie ahead.

A heart, imprinted

The most important component of a memory is the way it makes you feel.

It's that simple.

This thought has given me a lot of comfort lately: It isn't necessarily about *what* we do in our specific mothering journey, it is *how* we do the work that is the work itself.

I realized early on that I was not the best when it came to holidays (cue overnight delivery of Easter basket items from Amazon). But who is this for? My baby doesn't care if his wooden eggs are painted in the perfect pastel design. He would rather me just lie on the floor with him and tell an expressive story about how the Easter Bunny came to be (that I made up in the moment).

There is a lot they won't remember, and that we won't remember for that matter, but it's the way we make them *feel* that makes an imprint on their heart.

While we may never have all the answers, the way we show up each day is mothering in its most present form. It is all the moments in between, like when we are rocking our babies to sleep or making them snacks for the sixth time that day. These are the seeds of a childhood worth cherishing.

When our children look back, it won't be the perfectly curated details they'll recall. It will be the warmth of belonging, the feeling of being truly loved.

(A PRAYER FOR TODAY)

I ask that you give me grace in the moments when I feel the heavy weight of decisions on my shoulders. Help me convey my undying love for my child, no matter the occasion.

All mothers work

Motherhood is one of the most profound and transformative forms of work on this earth. "Work" is any mental, emotional, or physical effort undertaken to achieve a purpose—and what greater purpose exists than raising a child?

For a child to learn and grow, they need the foundation of feeling safe and valued. This foundation begins with you, Mama. You are creating the grounds for your child to flourish in life; you are watering them with love so their roots can grow deep and their branches wide.

It doesn't matter how the world chooses to label you—whether as a "stay-at-home mom" or a "working mom." The truth is simple: *all mothers work.* Every late night, every tear wiped away, every meal prepared, every hug given—this is work, sacred and purposeful.

So, next time you underestimate your value, remember that you are holding a world changer in your arms.

There is no greater work on this planet, and you were chosen for this role because no one else can do it like you. You are uniquely equipped, and you are living proof of the power of a mother's love.

You are doing the greatest work there is, Mama. Never forget that.

(A PRAYER FOR TODAY)

God, infuse my work as a mother with patience, love, and wisdom, filling each moment with grace and joy for my family. Help me remember my inherent worth and value to this world.

Sip of Self-Care:

The Sacredness in Small Things

It's easy to overlook the quiet work of motherhood—the crumbs wiped away, the tiny clothes folded, the gentle swaying to soothe a little one. These moments may seem small, but they carry immense weight. They are acts of love, threads weaving together the story of care and devotion you're creating.

Practice for Today:

As you wipe crumbs from the counter, pause for a moment and take a deep breath. Whisper to yourself: "This work is important."

While folding tiny clothes into neat stacks, let your fingers feel the softness of the fabric. Notice the care in each fold and repeat softly: "This work is important."

When you soothe a fizzy baby, swaying gently in the quiet, place your hand over your heart and remind yourself: "This work is important."

These seemingly ordinary tasks are the foundation of a home built on love and security. Every small act, every quiet moment, holds purpose and meaning. So, as you move through your day, carry this truth with you: *This work is important.*

And so are you.

You are the gatekeeper

In the early months of motherhood, I intentionally cleared out my schedule and was conscious about what I said yes to as I reentered the world. As the months went on, however, I slowly let my calendar and work obligations creep back up to pre-motherhood levels (essentially, I let my garden become overrun with weeds). This took an undeniable toll on me physically and mentally—I couldn't do it all.

Motherhood has taught me that I am not just the gatekeeper for who and what consumes my precious time and energy but also my child's. And it's now become one of the roles I take most seriously.

Saying no is a superpower—a deliberate act of pruning, creating space for the things your heart truly longs for.

You are the guardian of your family's time and energy, a role I've come to hold with deep reverence. I've realized that one of the greatest gifts I can give my child is the gift of simplicity: fewer plans, more blank space, and additional room to simply *be*. Sometimes, the kindest thing we can do as mothers is to say no, so we can protect the peace in our lives and cultivate a garden that blooms with intention.

(A PRAYER FOR TODAY)

God, give me the courage to say no with grace and kindness. May I tap into the wisdom within me that allows me to know when to open the gates and when to keep them closed.

All flowers need the rain

Maybe today is a bright day, or maybe it's one where you are struggling. All these days are necessary because they show you something about yourself.

When I became a mother, one feeling I was most surprised by was the anger I sometimes felt: anger at the world, at its pace, at the structural cracks in our society that make mothering harder instead of easier. Anger at the freedom my husband had or how many of the seemingly unimportant obligations, like ordering a bigger size of onesies or planning our next vacation, always fell on me. Anger at the way my friends or family would sometimes disappoint me. Anger at their lack of empathy or understanding. And let's be honest—feeling anger doesn't feel good. At its core, however, our feelings are information, and if we use it correctly, it can be a forcing function.

Holistic practitioner Dr. Erica Matluck, one of my dear friends, says that a mother's anger is actually a blessing to humanity when it serves as the emotional fuel to power the will of our solar plexus chakra (the energy center that governs our motivation).

When we feel a powerful emotion such as anger, we are more easily driven into action because we want to rid ourselves of the feeling and fix the problem. And if we can be driven into the right action, then our feelings can be the source of not only our own healing but also the healing of the collective.

So, the next time you feel anger, know that it can be a blessing, if only you use it as the fuel for change.

(A PRAYER FOR TODAY)

God, help me metabolize my anger into fuel for positive change, healing my heart and empowering me to make a lasting impact on the world.

Consistency is the key that you hold

Consistency is everything. We've heard this phrase as it relates to many things in our lives—health, work, sports, and even relationships. The same is true for our motherhood journey, but it takes on a whole new meaning in this context. It's not about doing the same practices every day or mastering any one of a number of routines. It's just about showing up. Every single day. And you do that for your baby.

It's our consistent presence they long for and what they need, *not perfection*. Knowing they can rely on us and always have someone in their corner is the key that unlocks their ability to feel safe and loved. We spend so much time trying to create the "perfect" childhood, but I felt a sigh of relief when I finally realized the moments they will remember most are those when we were there for them, holding their hands, kissing their boo-boos, and loving them in a way only a mother can do.

Some days I feel inspired to venture out into the world with my child. Other days, just stepping outside feels like a challenge. And that's okay. Life ebbs and flows, and so do we. Consistency doesn't mean doing everything the same way every day. It's about being present, through the highs and the lows, the energy-filled weeks and the quiet, stay-at-home ones. It's this simple truth: Your child doesn't need perfection; they just need *you*.

(A PRAYER FOR TODAY)

God, may I remember that I am consistent in my love and devotion to my baby like the steady flow of a river. Guide me through rough waters and calm steams so I remain steadfast in my efforts.

Grace—there is no sweeter gift

Take a look at yourself in the mirror. The woman you see is strong, sensitive, and kind. She is doing the best she can in every moment.

As mothers, we freely give grace to our children (rightfully so), to our partners (most of the time), and to our friends, but it is much harder to offer that same gift to ourselves. But here's the thing: Your little one is a mirror too. They notice how you interact with the world around you and that includes the way you treat and talk to yourself.

So, you owe it to yourself and your child to offer yourself grace every day from here on out. It can be as simple as saying I love you out loud to yourself or smiling at your reflection. It may sound silly, but it goes a long way in tending to the woman you are *becoming* and showing her how much you love her.

(A PRAYER FOR TODAY)

God, help me see myself the way you see me—full of kindness and love, radiating with beauty from the inside out. Guide my heart back to you over and over again when I am having a hard time finding the good within myself.

Sip of Self-Care:

A Silk-Wrapped Ritual for Rest

Before bed, create a soothing ritual to nurture yourself. Begin by gently massaging a small amount of castor oil onto your scalp or hairline, letting its warmth and richness seep in to nourish your hair and relax your mind. Then, wrap your hair in a soft silk head wrap, letting the smooth fabric cradle you in comfort as you prepare for rest.

Now, close your eyes and take three slow, deep breaths, allowing the day to melt away with each exhale. Between each breath, let a soft smile grace your lips. Feel your cheeks lift, the gentle warmth of the smile spreading across your face.

This smile is just for you—a quiet expression of gratitude and self-love. Imagine the silk wrap and castor oil working in tandem, not just caring for your hair but also symbolizing the care you deserve in every aspect of your life. As you drift off to sleep, carry this sense of comfort and ease into your dreams.

Healed people, heal people

When asked what the most important part of motherhood is, many would claim it's raising the child. But I would say, "It's healing the woman."

Healing ourselves is the most powerful thing we can do.

When a mother embarks on a journey of healing and self-discovery, she not only transforms her own life, but she also sends ripples of healing through generations.

When we heal ourselves, we become a soft and sturdy place for our children to land. We are nutrient-rich soil in which our children can take root and grow wildly.

As we tend to our own wounds with love and compassion, we model resilience and strength for our children and future generations.

A healed mother breaks patterns of pain and dysfunction, replacing them with seeds of empathy, understanding, and self-care.

A healed mother is attuned to her emotions and encourages her child to express their feelings in healthy ways, fostering emotional intelligence and resilience.

A healed mother fosters positive relationships with her child, partner, and others in her life. She is able to then model open communication and conflict resolution to create a nurturing and supportive environment in which her family can thrive.

A healed mother gifts her descendants with the invaluable legacy of emotional well-being, laying the foundation for a healthier and more harmonious future.

Be a healed mother. Whatever that takes, you deserve it, wholly. A healed mother changes the world because she heals those around her.

(A PRAYER FOR TODAY)

Infuse me with the strength and wisdom to embrace healing and emerge stronger, more whole, and entirely filled with your love.

Spiritual inheritance

When we think of the word "inheritance," our brain jumps to the tangible. But we inherit all kinds of things from the people in our lives, especially our parents. From physical characteristics to bad habits, there is much that is passed on from generation to generation. So, this got me thinking: What do I want my child to inherit from me from a spiritual perspective?

Of course, there will come a time when your child makes their own decisions as to what they believe in, but what do you want them to inherit (receive) from *you*? Whether we know it or not, we are handing something down, so we might as well be intentional about it.

When I was growing up, my parents made attending church a nonnegotiable part of life—Wednesdays and Sundays like clockwork. At the time, I resented it, or at least I thought I did.

As I grew up, however, I noticed that I felt at home in church. I loved the music and the way my spirits were lifted. In my hardest moments, I have turned to God. I inherited the idea that I was created by a good, loving, kind God from my parents, and it's something I want to pass on to my son. I want him to know there is a higher power, and that he is unconditionally loved.

I get to be the one who shows him what faith in God looks like—to have someone to turn to in difficult times and to thank for the blessings that adorn our lives. My beliefs may not mirror my parents' exactly, but the values they lived by are the threads that weave my own faith. My hope is that my child feels abundant in his spiritual inheritance, and my offering to him starts now.

(A PRAYER FOR TODAY)

God, it is imperative that my child is introduced to you. Thank you for your unwavering promise to love my baby and care for them long after I am gone. May the seed of your presence that I plant grow throughout their lifetime so they will aways have peace and a belief system.

Good stress also exists

Believe it or not, not all stress is bad. In fact, we need some level of it to survive. It's as central to our well-being as air, in the right doses. I invite you to start thinking of stress as simply a natural biological response to the stimulation of demands. Think of it like a signal or alarm that is meant to tell us important information and that can be divided into two categories: healthy stress and unhealthy stress.

Unhealthy stress is the kind most of us are referring to when we use the term. This type of stress lets us know when the demands on our time, energy, and attention have gotten to be *too much*. It comes from simply pushing through without awareness about how uncomfortable we are. In this state, we may miss the chance to identify the root cause because we are operating from a place of instability and overload. Healthy stress, on the other hand—when the demands create a helpful invitation, essentially stimulating without overstimulating us—can motivate us to adapt to challenges in our lives. The truth is that without this kind of stress, we would never grow.

So, the first step in stress management is simply to begin recognizing the difference. Is this stress *for* you or *against* you? There will surely be times in motherhood when you feel overwhelmed. How can you begin seeing the feelings that arise as information you use as a tool to your well-being? Maybe you need to lessen your workload; perhaps you can distance yourself from certain people/projects. Or perhaps you are feeling unmotivated and need to create more stimulation, newness, or adventure in your life. Maybe you need to step out of your comfort zone.

The next time you feel stressed, start to get curious.

(A PRAYER FOR TODAY)

God, help me find the right balance of demands on my time and attention so that I may remain grounded but also inspired. May I have the courage to find the right balance, experimenting with adding and subtracting the load on my body, mind, and spirit.

Honor your many versions

Sometimes I look in the mirror and can't believe how much I have changed. Other times, I feel stagnant.

But just as you can't see your hair growing millimeter by millimeter, your metamorphosis is happening right now, often under the radar.

As the saying goes, "The days are long, but the years are short." This reality has never been more apparent than now. Daily routines meld together, yet I can't seem to convince time to be on my side. I recently bought wooden milestone markers to capture my baby at every thirty-day milestone, and my stomach drops each time I realize we are already overdue. You, too, may be wondering how you are already almost three hundred days into motherhood.

It feels like we are in a hurry to get to the next thing, the next moment, the next milestone, or even the next daily chore. It's only when we take a pause that we realize how much time has already passed, how much forward movement is occurring.

So today, let's explore how we can stretch into this pause.

Can you bring awareness to your breath? Can you tune into the sensations of being in the present moment with this version of you and your little one?

The present moment is truly all that we have. This version of you is like a fleeting rainbow—beautiful, ephemeral, and gone before we know it. See her, embrace her, and cherish her while she stands before you.

(A PRAYER FOR TODAY)

God, in the stillness of this moment, I pause to honor the many versions of myself that have come and gone. Help me to see the beauty in the fleeting seasons of my life, just as I marvel at the growth of my little one.

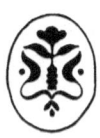

Sip of Self-Care:

Blooming through Breath

Try meditation in its simplest form—by following your breath. Inhale, exhale. When your mind starts to wander (as it naturally will), gently bring it back to your breath without judgment.

Now, add a touch of creativity to your practice: Imagine each wandering thought as the beginning of a petal being drawn, and as you return to your breath, the petal line is completed. With each return, another petal is added, forming your unique flower.

Remember, meditation isn't about creating a "perfect" flower. Your blooms may have petals of all shapes and sizes, reflecting the beauty of your practice. Whether your meditation lasts one minute or ten, know that each moment spent with your breath adds to the vibrant garden within you.

Try this today—breathe, wander, return, and bloom. See how it feels to nurture yourself, one petal at a time.

Have patience with the process

Coffee is everywhere, on every corner and in many cupboards. And like most things in life, we see the finished product without often thinking about the process involved.

A coffee bean has an incredible story though. It begins inside the cherry of a coffee plant, (yes, a cherry—the coffee bean is actually a seed equivalent to a cherry pit). The cherries are then handpicked by skilled farmers who wait for the perfect moment: too soon, and the bean is sour; too late, and it risks decay. Not all ripen at once, so farmers must return to the same plant again and again, carefully selecting only those ready for harvest.

From there, the beans are extracted from the cherries and laid out to dry under the sun's warmth. Once dried, they undergo the hulling process where the outer layers of parchment and mucilage are removed to reveal the green coffee beans inside. Finally, the beans are sent to the roasters where they undergo a transformative process, as heat coaxes out the rich, aromatic oils that define their unique flavor.

So why am I telling you this? I believe we, as mothers, can glean important lessons from this journey:

- Patience is key. Growth happens on its own schedule. Just as cherries ripen at different times, every child—and every mother—is on their own path. Let go of comparison and embrace your unique season.

- Every stage serves a purpose. The trials, hardships, and moments of joy are all shaping you, just as each step transforms the bean into coffee. What looks simple from the outside, rarely is. Behind every perfect cup is a long, intricate process we often overlook.

So today, Mama, savor your coffee. Let each sip be a reminder of the extraordinary journey from plant to palate. And know that your transformative journey of matrescence is also underway.

(A PRAYER FOR TODAY)

May I see the value in the hard moments that have led me to this point. May I have patience in your process as we co-create this version of my life in motherhood.

A note on timelines

The best advice I have ever been given in motherhood is this: You can have it all, just not necessarily all at the same time. Those words landed deeply within me, shifting my perspective in profound ways. I was a multifaceted, multi-passionate human being before becoming a mother. And I still am. For so much of this past year, I have been searching, trying to figure out who I am in this new role. Varying parts of me feel muted, and some of the career aspirations I had no longer feel important.

Right now, I am loving being in the feminine energy of motherhood, so I have spent hours contemplating what that means. Are those other parts of me gone forever? Has the fire to achieve them died? For me, I have decided that those aspirations I once had are still alive within me like a slow burning ember, but some of them are not meant to be a part of the season I am in *right now*. I may have the fuel to fan that flame later, but it's not now. And that's okay.

Whether it's career choices, friendships, hobbies, or any other part of your life before your baby, know that just because you take a break doesn't mean it's gone. Harvest what is ripe this season and trust that the rest will remain, tucked safely beneath the surface, waiting for you when the time is right.

(A PRAYER FOR TODAY)

As I journey through life's ebbs and flows, grant me the wisdom to find balance in all aspects of my being. Help me harmonize my responsibilities with moments of rest, my ambitions with moments of gratitude, and my challenges with moments of resilience.

The rainbow of motherhood

Today, my son saw his first rainbow. Did you know rainbows are actually full circles? From the ground, we only see half, but from above—like in an airplane—you can glimpse their wholeness. God's designs never cease to amaze me.

And no two rainbows are exactly alike. The appearance of each one is dependent on the size of the raindrops, the angle of the sunlight, and the observer's position, making each rainbow a unique display of nature. The perfect alchemy of water and sunlight.

Each rainbow, like motherhood, is completely unique, shaped by its conditions, yet undeniably beautiful. Motherhood, too, is a vivid spectrum: the passionate reds of love and protection, the bright yellows of joy, the soft greens of growth, and the deep blues of calm. And just as rainbows emerge after rain, motherhood's most radiant colors often follow moments of challenge. Wherever you are on this arc today, know that you are not alone in your journey, and remember that the rain always comes first. So, embrace those moments that feel difficult, for they will give way to the radiant colors of your journey.

The treasure to be found is not at the end or the destination but rather in the witnessing. It is in the recognition of beauty in the glimmers of sunlight reflected from theirs to yours and back again.

Open your eyes and see the beauty. Let it take your breath away, time and time again, Mama.

(A PRAYER FOR TODAY)

May I find hope in every low moment, just as the rainbow follows the storm. Guide me to cherish the vibrant spectrum of experiences and to trust that your light will always shine through, illuminating my path with your boundless love and promise.

You are growing, even on days it doesn't feel like it

Motherhood resembles a blooming flower, infusing the garden of life with vivid colors of love, care, and fulfillment in ways I didn't know was possible. Similar to how the sun's rays foster the growth of seeds, the journey of motherhood cultivates a profound sense of connection with all of the seemingly scattered parts of ourselves and others, in the nature that surrounds us, and in the humanity that dots the earth. Amid the storms of trials and the gentle rain of happiness, we uncover a deep well of inner fortitude, perseverance, and self-awareness that turns us upside down entirely.

Today, while driving, my son began to cry. I played a soft, reassuring song and gently reminded him he was safe, that we were nearly there. In that small moment, I paused and recognized how far I'd come. I thought back to Day 69 in this book—the last time something similar happened, I was the one pulling over in tears!

We are not static in this transformation. Far from it.

Motherhood moves us, shifts us, and rewrites us completely. It unravels every thread of who we were only to weave those threads into an entirely new design, a pattern richer and more intricate than we could have imagined.

This is the journey. This is motherhood.

(A PRAYER FOR TODAY)

God, in this sacred moment, I ask that you remind me of the immense growth and expansion I am experiencing. Just as a seedling pushes through the soil, reaching toward the nourishing sunlight, help me recognize my own strength and resilience as I navigate the challenges and joys of embracing my role as a mother.

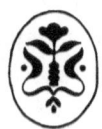

Sip of Self-Care:

Grounding through Touch: A Simple Practice for Overwhelming Moments

Take a moment to connect with yourself through the simple, grounding act of touch. Begin by gently pressing the pad of your thumb on each hand to the tips of your other fingers, one by one. Move slowly and intentionally, noticing the texture, warmth, and sensation of your skin.

This small but powerful action brings you back to the present moment, offering a sense of calm amid the thrill and overwhelm of motherhood. As you connect with your fingertips, remind yourself: *Everything I need is already within me.*

You can return to this practice anytime you feel anxious or untethered. Let the simplicity of touch anchor you in the here and now, a quiet reminder of your strength and resourcefulness.

All shadows are created from a beacon of light

The term "shadow" has an implicit negative tone to it, an unwanted darkness. But have you looked at your shadow lately? I caught mine (or rather "ours" as my baby was at my hip) the other day as we walked along the lake, his coos bringing a gentle smile to my face. Three things struck me about our silhouettes dancing upon the canvas of the concrete wall:

One, you only have a shadow when your life is full of sunshine. I thought about the various parts of life that feel light-filled right now. For me, it's peaceful mornings with my baby; walking outside and smiling at the flurry of squirrels that make him laugh; the tender rediscovery of connection as my husband and I nurture our marriage.

Two, there's a quiet comfort in the consistency of your shadow appearing. You don't have to work for it or wonder whether it will show up; it's a given. It's a gentle reminder that even in the background, your influence as a mother is always there providing love, guidance, and support.

Three, as I lifted my hand and waved to my own reflection in the concrete, my son raised his as well. To me, this so beautifully depicts why we do what we do. No matter how hard this journey gets, no matter how many tears we wipe away or messes we clean up, no matter what changes our body endures, to have those little shadows following after us, mimicking our words, loving us so fully that they search for our face among the rest, makes it all worthwhile.

May your shadows remind you of all of this—that your life is full of sun, that your unwavering presence is felt so deeply, and that in your reflection, your baby is there, watching you with eyes of wonder and awe.

In your shadow is warmth and light. A mother's love, a beacon bright.

(A PRAYER FOR TODAY)

Thank you for sending this little being into my life to teach me, expand me, and initiate me into a deeper love than I ever knew was possible.

Know that you can adjust course

Family can be a beautiful mirror, but it can also feel like a minefield of unresolved tensions, old wounds, and well-meaning but uninvited opinions. As Ram Dass said, "If you think you're enlightened, go spend a week with your family."[13]

And when you bring a new baby into the mix, you're navigating both family dynamics and their interactions with your child. Maybe your siblings or parents overstep, give unsolicited advice, or disregard your parenting preferences. It's a tightrope walk between standing up for your values as a mother and keeping the peace as a sister and daughter, knowing the visit is only temporary.

It's hard. When someone interferes with your carefully chosen parenting approach, it can feel like an unspoken challenge to your role. And let's face it, there's no handbook for how to respond. I'm not here to tell you to "just let it go," nor am I suggesting you always "take a stand." What I want you to know is this: family relationships are complex, and you'll be navigating these waters for years to come.

If you try one approach and it doesn't sit well with you, adjust course next time. If something weighs heavy on your heart, confide in your partner or a trusted family member to come up with a plan. The beauty of this journey is that you *can* do things differently. You have every right to steer your family life in the way that feels true to you.

(A PRAYER FOR TODAY)

God, in moments of struggle, I lift up my heart to you. Please give me the wisdom to handle things with patience and grace. May I see my loved ones through your eyes so I can communicate with kindness and hold on to the hope that we will find a way through.

Meditate in the mess

I walked into a Mommy and Me baby yoga class and sat down. The teacher was warm and inviting as she reassured us that it was a judgment-free zone and noted that our baby crying was often more upsetting to us than to anyone else in the class. She said that the point of the class was just to learn to find our breath and meet ourselves where we were. And then she said something that has stuck with me since that day: "Remember, you can take this practice of mindfulness and breath with you anywhere you go, and you should always feel empowered to meditate in the mess."

Easier said than done for sure because if you're anything like me, it's hard to close my eyes and drop in when the dishes are piling up or there are toys on the floor. But if we let those things constantly delay our meditation, then we will never get there. So today, I invite you to let go of expectations of perfection and allow yourself to simply be.

Meditating in the mess means finding stillness and calm *amid the chaos*, nurturing your inner peace and resilience. What a power, what a gift we can cultivate—the ability to anchor in, regardless of what swirls outside of us. Remember, you deserve moments of tranquility, and peace can be found even in the busiest of days. Meditate in the mess.

(A PRAYER FOR TODAY)

God, give me peace amid the mess, where I can quiet my mind and reconnect to my inner landscape. Guide me in weaving moments of meditation into the fabric of my daily life, so that I may find clarity, renewal, and strength to face whatever challenges come my way.

Fear is just information

When I was pregnant, I was working as an in-house lawyer for a large and prestigious nonprofit. As I prepared to go on maternity leave, I had a deep-seated fear that I would be "left behind" in my career as a working mother. I was afraid of losing myself and the life that I had worked so hard to create. Who was I without adding value?

My identity felt tied to my career. To make matters worse, my counterpart in the office was a good friend but also a male in his thirties without a care in the world. It wasn't until I had my son that I had the space to really sit with these fears, and in doing so, they became my guide. I realized how much I loved some aspects of my work, but there were other aspects that I was ready to move on from. My fear became the compass I needed to find my next position, one that gave me the same fulfillment but with more flexibility. My wounded inner child told me I needed to stay stagnant in my previous role for notoriety, but once healed, I felt empowered to reach out to my network and find the job that's right for me now, *in this season.*

Fear can be scary, of course, but it can also be a gift. Fear is information from which we can gain knowledge. It reveals the truth, if we let it. Fear is simply our courage becoming known.

(A PRAYER FOR TODAY)

God, open my heart and mind to what you are trying to tell me. Let my fears reveal the path forward and allow me the courage to take the first step despite those fears.

Sip of Self-Care:

Journal or ponder on these questions today:

- What is a fear that loops in my mind or holds me captive?
- Where does that fear live in my body?
- What information is this fear trying to tell me?

Stand tall as a mother

Standing tall in your confidence as a mother is a deeply rooted belief in your abilities and worthiness as a parent. It means embracing your unique strengths, instincts, and experiences to make decisions for you and your child.

One of your strengths can be found in the knowledge and inner knowing you have about what is in the best interest of your baby. This doesn't mean that you are perfect or that your decisions are always right, but it does mean you are resilient and adaptable, you seek support when you need it, you shake off mistakes when made, and you continue your evolution as the mother.

I recently had a playdate with a friend. She had only been at my house for about forty-five minutes when her little one started to cry. My friend stood up and confidently declared, "We need to head out. He is tired and really needs a good nap at home." They quickly packed up and said their goodbyes.

As she drove away, I reflected on my friend's ability to read her child and confidently advocate for him. I wasn't offended by her sudden departure, or that our date was cut short. I was honestly inspired. And empowered. Because when we speak our truth, we give a nod to those around us that it's safe to do the same in their lives as well.

She knew what needed to be done, and she did it. It was as simple as that. Your love runs wide and deep, so stand tall in your abilities as an empowered mother. And it's empowered mothers that we need, our children need, and the world needs.[14]

(A PRAYER FOR TODAY)

God, help me tether to my inner knowing and speak up for myself and my child. May I stand tall in my worthiness as a mother and feel confident that I am the best equipped (even when it doesn't feel like it) to know what my child needs in any given moment.

Expect the best from God

Have you ever had something happen that you didn't understand? Of course you have. For me, that something was getting pregnant.

I knew I wanted children, but when I took that pregnancy test offhandedly while using the restroom between Zoom meetings (this was early COVID, and I clearly felt emboldened with my newfound freedom to multitask), I was shocked.

It actually took me four days to tell my husband. Not because I was upset, but because it just didn't feel real. I couldn't picture my life with a child, and I needed to have some conversations with God before I was ready to share the news.

I look back at that moment now and giggle to myself. Of course I was ready (as ready as I would have ever been). Of course it was the right time (as right as it would have ever been).

And it has been the biggest earth-shattering, life-changing miracle I could have ever imagined. But I couldn't see it then because unlike God, we aren't privy to the larger schematic plan that makes up our life.

Remember that life and God are working *for you*, not against you. In the moments when we don't understand why things are unfolding the way they are, we can be assured that God's hand is working, guiding us down a path that will lead to more blessings than we hope for.

Expect the best. It's what is coming your way, Mama.

(A PRAYER FOR TODAY)

God, I come to you with an expectant heart, believing in your goodness to bring forth the best outcomes in every aspect of my life.

There is a lot of noise out there, so turn up the volume of your own voice

What is it like inside your head? It may sound like a strange question, but really, pause for a moment and try to answer it. Is it loud? Does it hum with your voice or the echoes of others? Is the voice kind to you? What does she sound like?

Thinking is sometimes an endless conversation, often with yourself as both speaker and listener. But when we are thinking all the time, there is no space left for listening—to the world around us, to others, or even to our own deeper wisdom. My dad, who was always the quiet type, often reminds me that listening is one of the most overlooked skill sets. He didn't say much, but when he did, you knew it came from a place of intention and depth. I used to wonder if his silence wasn't silence at all but a kind of stillness where real listening happens.

In our own minds, we can cultivate that same stillness. I like to imagine our inner world as a DJ console, with dials and sliders to control the volume, tempo, and rhythm of the thoughts that play on repeat. We can turn down the external tracks—the noise of the world, the chatter of distractions—and make room for something softer to emerge.

It's in that quiet that we can hear the melody of our authentic self, the rhythm of our inner wisdom.

This harmonious mix is soft to the ears and sweet to the soul, and it's where we can find clarity, purpose, power, and freedom to dance to the rhythm of our authentic self amid the bustling noise of the world's stage.

(A PRAYER FOR TODAY)

Silence the noise of the world so that I may hear the downloads you give me and the pings that you send to my heart and soul.

Recycle and reuse

As a meditation guide, I sometimes cue my students to imagine anything heavy, sad, or challenging that lives within their mind and body as withering leaves that they can gather and push into a big pile. I then invite them to send that pile down and out of the body and into the earth.

One day after a session, a student mentioned they felt guilty sending such heavy energy from the "ugly" or hard parts of their lives to the beautiful earth.

But that's not the way it works. Because the earth sees it all as *neutral*.

It's our human experience that puts the labels of "good" or "bad" onto them. These experiences, feelings, and situations are negative to us alone. When we send that energy down and out of the body, we are sending it to be recycled and reused elsewhere.

The earth can take it. The earth can transform it.

Any challenge you've been through (or are currently going through), no matter how difficult, can be composted into the fertile soil in which new life can grow.

(A PRAYER FOR TODAY)

I offer up the hard experiences as compost for growth. Transform the pain and challenges that exist in my life into nourishment for my soul. Help me see the beauty that arises from adversity and use it to cultivate brighter days ahead.

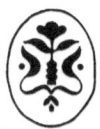

Sip of Self-Care:

The practice of forest bathing can be incredibly healing—and no, it doesn't even involve water! It involves immersing yourself in nature, particularly in forests, to experience the therapeutic benefits of being surrounded by trees, fresh air, and natural sounds. It has various health benefits such as improved mood, reduced stress levels, and enhanced immune function. Begin by finding a local area where you can walk among nature, stopping to listen to the sounds of the birds and taking in the beauty.

Can you slow down to really notice using your five senses? Can you release any heavy energy and breathe in the vitality that surrounds you? That's forest bathing!

Your baby as a sovereign being

A dear friend of mine is a Human Design reader. If you aren't familiar with this concept, there are five different types of human designs that you could be based on the date, time, and place of your birth, and it incorporates astrology as well as other frameworks (I encourage you to look yours up!).

We had her do a reading for my son, and it was so interesting to hear the results.

It turns out he is a "Projector" and is one who requires more down time to recharge his energy. I, on the other hand, am a "Generator," which means I can generate energy easily. We couldn't be more opposite in that way, and it got me thinking. Just because our children come from us doesn't mean they are the *same* as us.

Maybe they will have shared interests with us as they age, but maybe not.

Maybe they have physical characteristics that resemble us, but maybe not.

Maybe they will have our mannerisms, but maybe not.

Because at the end of the day, they are still their own sovereign beings.

This seems obvious, but when we spend ten months being in one body and then the next twelve months carrying them on our hip, doing whatever we do, it's easy to forget.

So, take time today just to observe and appreciate things you already notice that differ from you. And whether the concept of Human Design is something that interests you or not, I encourage you to seek frameworks that may shed light on who your baby is at their core. Especially during these first few years when our babies cannot express themselves fully with words, how can we take an interest in their idiosyncrasies? How can we honor the sovereign beings they are?

(A PRAYER FOR TODAY)

Help me gather little pearls of wisdom about my baby's budding personality so that I can better help them bloom brightly according to the way you designed them.

Your most expansive self

Expand into your initiation, Mama.

One day at a time. Looking back at when you first brought your little angel earthside almost a year ago, to now, this present day in time. So much has changed. So fast and yet so slowly.

The initiation of motherhood can feel like a whirlwind of hormones and emotions. Dreams and desires. On some days you'll feel the urge to contract, to retreat into yourself. Other days, you'll feel the pull to expand, to stretch your capacity, your abilities, your patience, your love, your commitment, and the depth in who you are becoming. It's the rhythm of the inhale *and* the exhale, an ebb and a flow. The ease and the effort.

Motherhood has room for your ambitious self, but perhaps it will be a softer and fuller version. Let this new version of you unfold with grace.

(A PRAYER FOR TODAY)

God, guide me, lead me into my next expansion. I am ready, I am willing. I am here. With every passing day, and each moment, may my heart, my love, my capacity, and my wisdom expand.

Lead with a soft heart and strong boundaries

You get to set the standards, Mama. Everywhere you go. With everyone you meet. In every interaction.

Your boundaries set the tone for how you want your relationships, friendships, and motherhood to flow, to align, to be witnessed and respected. And in setting these boundaries, you create a container of peace around your whole family unit. The free-flowing advice on social media, the drama in your extended family, the gossip in your friend group, the rumors floating around the office—none deserve a place in your house, either physically or metaphorically. Where in your life do you need to refine your standards and honor them—for you, for your baby, for your family?

Early on, I had friends who wanted to spend time with me but didn't take much interest in my baby. In the beginning, I told myself that it was okay, as not everyone is a "kid person." But the more I sat with it, the more it bothered me. My baby *is* me in many ways. For some of these relationships, I spoke up about how I was feeling. For others, I let them take their natural course.

You set the tone for your motherhood to flourish and thrive in ways only you can know. And you are allowed to outgrow relationships and priorities that are no longer aligned. Tune into the places and spaces that disrupt your peace. Start distancing yourself from those people, places, and things. Notice whether your peace grows.

(A PRAYER FOR TODAY)

Today, I ask for the strength to build walls where I need them and the courage to protect my time and energy for myself and for my baby. Help me find the right balance so I can take care of myself and be the best mom I can be. Fill my heart with your love and light and give me the clarity to create a peaceful, balanced life.

Rewilding motherhood

What is it about things that are wild that make them so endearing?

I think of the beauty of wildflowers or the difference between seeing a bird caged in the zoo versus watching it soar high against the blue sky above my head.

What makes being wild so attractive is that it's *free and unpredictable*, and therefore, it has an element of mystery about it. It's true to its essence without trying to conform to anything around it.

When an environmentalist seeks to rewild land, it entails returning it to its natural state—vibrant and free.

I invite you to reclaim your motherhood journey in the same way, returning to your true soul essence of who *you* are as a mother. Not bound by rules or expectations, but instead free-flowing, unpredictable, and deeply rooted in love and spirituality. Let the grounds of your journey be nourished by what matters most to you, your truth, your instincts, your connection to God. And let it grow wild from there, untamed in every direction.

Embrace the unpredictable nature that makes the initiation of matrescence uniquely yours.

(A PRAYER FOR TODAY)

God, please keep my motherhood journey wild, filled with unexpected adventures, untamed love, and joyful spontaneity as we navigate life's beautiful chaos together.

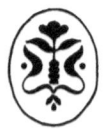

Sip of Self-Care:

Pick a day this week to do something different with your baby than you have ever done before. Take a surprise picnic, an unplanned road trip to a flower field nearby, or a hike that you have been wanting to try. Go into it knowing that there may be hiccups, but let that be okay. The fun is in the spontaneity. Give yourself permission to keep the planning down to a minimum, then see how it all unfolds. Let it surprise you!

You don't have to value what the world does

Economics teaches us that every choice comes with an opportunity cost—trade-offs shaped by what we value most.

But in motherhood, these decisions become infinitely more layered. The opportunity cost of going back to work or taking on more hours means sacrificing precious time with our children.

Yet, this doesn't mean we value motherhood any less than our careers. Instead, it reflects the constraints of the societal framework we operate within.

Society has determined the going rate for sitting behind a desk or in front of a computer, and surprise, it's higher than the going rate for mothering our children, which is zero.

I am still not quite sure how this rate was determined, since mothering is objectively holy.

As mothers, we soothe another person when they are crying. We hold space for their emotional development. We are caring for the *most* vulnerable subset of our population: our babies.

I see this truth clearly. I feel it deeply. And I know you do too.

So, the next time you feel like you're making an impossible decision, remember to extend yourself grace. You're navigating a system that was never designed to honor what truly matters. Whatever path you choose, or your circumstances dictate, let it be rooted in love, the unwavering currency of motherhood. It's what fuels every decision, every sacrifice, every cherished moment.

And that love? It's beyond value. It's priceless.

(A PRAYER FOR TODAY)

Grant me the wisdom to listen into my heart's call for how I spend my days. Give me peace and ease as I navigate the tricky terrain of working and mothering at the same time. Also, please send me the lottery numbers when you have a moment.

The metamorphosis of motherhood

As you know, a caterpillar undergoes the most intense metamorphosis. This stage is so transformative that the caterpillar's body breaks down and reorganizes into a completely new being. A whole new sense of existence. On the other side of the cocoon, the butterfly has to work and struggle to break through, a test nature intentionally plays to strengthen its wings for flight. Finally, the butterfly emerges and stretches its wings, feeling the rush of life in a form it never knew, ready to soar into the sky and explore the world with newfound freedom.

Motherhood is very much like that cocoon. It changes you, transforms you into a whole new version of yourself. Your most powerful version is birthed through this initiation, bringing forth strength, grace, and power you didn't think was possible. The sleepless nights, the overwhelming emotions, the moments of doubt and uncertainty—they are all part of your metamorphosis.

Every challenge you face, every tear you shed, every ounce of love you pour out is contributing to your transformation. You are growing, expanding, and *becoming*. You are discovering depths of resilience and reservoirs of love that you never knew existed. Like the butterfly strengthening its wings to break free, every struggle in your journey prepares you to rise.

Now, it's your time to lift your wings toward the heavens and take flight— stronger, braver and more radiant than ever before.

(A PRAYER FOR TODAY)

God, transform me into the channel I am here to be. Transform me into the mother I am meant to be. Transform my heart, my soul, my body, and my mind.

You are raising the next generation

Every day that you get up and love on your baby, you are doing the most important work in the world because you are raising the next generation of changemakers and world shakers. When we love and care for our babies in this way, we are allowing them to feel safe and supported, which is the foundation for confident humans who can trust and love others.

You have the most loving heart and the softest embrace, and you are the fiercest protector of all your loved ones.

Your body is a beautiful sacred haven of nourishment and strength.

Your soul holds the language and codes of your ancestors. You know how to do this thing called motherhood. It's in your DNA. Tune out the noise and attune to the voice of God, of your soul, of your body.

So, every time you start to feel murky in the mundane, just know that your love makes a difference in this world, Mama.

(A PRAYER FOR TODAY)

God, thank you for your unwavering trust in me to shepherd the next generation. May I always feel you guiding me so that I can do my part in guiding my baby into the person they are meant to be.

The beauty of unplugging

A friend once reminded me that everything functions a little better after it's been unplugged and plugged back in, and that includes you, Mama.

We all need a reset. Maybe it's on a weekly basis or maybe it's daily, but we all need it eventually or else we risk burning out our internal circuit (which takes much longer to recover from than if we proactively detach from what is requiring our energy). When we spend even a microcosm of time "unplugged" or disconnected from the chaos of the outside world, we break that connection between our mind and all that is swirling around in our lives.

In doing so, we offer ourselves the chance to begin again.

And that feels so good. It's a new beginning with a fresh slate.

(A PRAYER FOR TODAY)

God, I ask you to help me separate from distractions and instead cultivate moments of peace and rejuvenation in my daily existence. Allow me to fully engage with my baby from a place of love as I cherish the sweet and fleeting memories that we are making here and now.

Sip of Self-Care:

Unplug and Nourish: A Kitchen Reset

Step into the kitchen, leave your phone behind, and bake a simple, postpartum-friendly treat that will fill your home with warmth and comfort: Banana Oat Cookies. These cookies are quick, nourishing, and perfect for busy moments.

INGREDIENTS:

- 2 ripe bananas, mashed
- 1 cup rolled oats
- 2 tbsp almond butter (or any nut/seed butter)
- 1/4 tsp cinnamon
- A handful of dark chocolate chips or dried fruit (optional)

INSTRUCTIONS:

1. Preheat your oven to 350°F (175°C) and line a baking sheet with parchment paper.
2. In a bowl, mix the mashed bananas, oats, almond butter, and cinnamon until well combined. Fold in chocolate chips or dried fruit if desired.
3. Scoop small spoonfuls of the mixture onto the baking sheet and gently flatten into cookie shapes.
4. Bake for 12–15 minutes, or until the edges are golden.

As the cookies bake, let the cozy aroma fill your space. Take a moment to breathe deeply and enjoy the pause.

When they're ready, savor a warm cookie fresh from the oven, letting its sweetness remind you of the small joys you deserve. This isn't just about baking, it's about nourishing your body, calming your mind, and creating a comforting space for you and your little one.

A note on strength

I recently tried a cold plunge for the first time and barely lasted thirty seconds. I felt deflated. There was a stranger next to me, and as we got to talking, I mentioned that I had a small baby. He turned to me and said, "If you have a baby, then this pales in comparison to what you've done in birthing a child."

I felt a lot of pride in that moment. And he was right. I have reached the end of my physical, mental, and emotional limits many times over these past ten months. Yet I'm still standing. Still showing up. Still moving forward.

Truly, though, is there anyone or anything stronger than a mother?

There is no clocking out, no quitting; there are no sick days or paid vacations. You can't walk away when things get hard. You can cry, but only for a moment because you will inevitably soon be needed. You can have bad days, but you still show up despite them. Your shoulders never give out. And you can even hold your pee for an insanely long period of time. You are so strong, Mama.

You should use this strength as a constant reminder that if you can do all this, you can do *anything*. So, the next time you doubt yourself, remember your strength. No one else could do it quite like you.

(A PRAYER FOR TODAY)

God, help me remember that I have endless strength to nurture and guide my baby with love and grace. Empower me to overcome every challenge that comes my way, no matter how big or small it may seem to others around me.

You are a somatic being

There is a profound wisdom within your body—more than any book, video, or theory could ever teach. Your body knows the way. It speaks to you in sensations, emotions, and impulses long before your conscious mind can catch up.

Have you ever met someone (a friend/partner) and your heart became immediately open? Have you ever encountered a person and felt chills because their energy was off? We are somatic beings. Our senses can pick up on things that our brain takes time to catch up to consciously. The question is, will we listen? How do we respond to the pings and messages that our body is sending? The more we spend time with our body, the more we recognize her voice.

For a long time, I felt disconnected from this truth. I approached movement, like yoga, with the mindset that its purpose was to sculpt my body. If I couldn't *see* the change, I felt like I wasn't getting enough out of it. But after giving birth, I rediscovered the deeper intention of the practice. Yoga is not about aesthetics, it's about coming home to yourself. The term "yoga" comes from a Sanskrit word meaning "to yoke" or "to unite." In essence, yoga brings your body and mind into alignment so they can communicate with clarity and ease.

Maybe yoga isn't your path, maybe it's some other form of movement. Any movement that allows you to inhabit your body fully is an opportunity to receive its messages. When we move, we bring ourselves into union with our deepest selves, and with God.

(A PRAYER FOR TODAY)

God, help me tune into the vessel that you have given me, my body, so I hear the messages that come from my heart, gut, and soul in addition to those directly from you.

You are magic

I say this with all my heart: while you may be replaceable in many aspects of life, whether at work or in other roles, you are absolutely *irreplaceable* in your role as mother. No one does it like you. A mother's love and presence cannot be replicated. You encompass an alchemy of warmth and depth that no one else does. By now you may even have concrete examples of it. Perhaps you notice that when your baby is crying, they stop the moment someone hands them to you.

I began to understand this once my baby spent time with my parents. They were wonderful, of course, but most of the time, it was my touch, my love, my way of being, that soothed my baby the best. It's a bond that is unique to the two of us.

And remember, seeking help and support doesn't take away from this magic, it only allows you to rest and recharge, which ultimately benefits both you and your little one.

While this may be exhausting at times, especially when you long for some help, like at night, it's also one of your superpowers.

Never forget the power you wield. You truly are magic, Mama.

(A PRAYER FOR TODAY)

God, thank you for the love you have placed in my heart as the mother of my child. Help me cherish and honor this special gift, recognizing its enduring beauty and strength in shaping my heart and soul.

Life, interrupted

If I'm honest, the root of my most frequent frustration in motherhood is the constant start and stop. Let me be clear: I don't view my baby as a bother. It's the challenge of dealing with my own unfinished tasks, the way something as simple as meal prep or writing can stretch out longer than it used to, or how it feels impossible to complete anything without interruption.

I jump in the shower, then my baby wakes up early from a nap.

I start a project, then my baby wants to be rocked.

I sit down to write, then my baby needs to be fed.

I don't think I am alone in this. It's the one thing that sets the mother–child relationship apart from all others. The dynamic between a mother and child is unlike any other because mothering means being available, often at a moment's notice. If my husband interrupted me every time I sat down to eat a meal or have a moment of peace—urgently, no less—I imagine we'd have some serious tension. But with motherhood, it's different. These interruptions aren't just expected, they're necessary. They are the rhythms of nurturing a dependent little one, helping them grow and feel secure in the world.

It's a natural part of the job if we are living our lives *and* being the sun around which our baby's world revolves (although it often feels the other way around). So, the question isn't how we stop the interruptions but rather how we can *shift* our perspective on them.

I've begun thinking of these interruptions as detours, not disturbances. Just like detours always lead you to your destination—albeit by a different route—it comforts me to know that I'll still get where I'm going. These detours aren't setbacks. In motherhood, they are simply part of the journey, gently reminding us that both the big moments and the small ones, like taking a shower, are worth honoring along the way, even if it takes a little longer than expected to get there.

(A PRAYER FOR TODAY)

God, please help me remember that my baby's needs aren't intentional disruptions but minor detours that will always return me to the path I'm meant to be on.

Sip of Self-Care:

Complete something today. It can be as simple as a promise you made to yourself. Enjoy a full cup of coffee, slowly. Call a friend. Take the first step in launching your new business idea (like buying the website domain). It's not about how big the gesture is, it's about holding yourself to finishing something you set out to do.

No matter what, I am your home

When we think of home, we tend to think of a place, one that provides safety, warmth, and shelter. But what if home were a person?

Well, for your baby, that person is you, Mama.

You are your baby's sanctuary, their place of refuge and safety in a world of unknowns. They are deeply cherished and loved in your arms, both physically and emotionally. You are the lullabies they hear in the quiet of the night and the gentle whispers of encouragement that accompany every milestone and sweet moment they experience.

Our love creates a foundation of trust and belonging so our babies can freely express themselves and explore the wonders of this earth with the knowledge we are always there, steadfast in our devotion to them.

You are someone's home, their strong foundation. What a beautiful responsibility. Hold it with confidence and care.

(A PRAYER FOR TODAY)

God, help me realize that I am my child's home, a sanctuary of love, safety, and unwavering support. Guide me as I nurture my little one with warmth and grace, guiding them through life's journey with compassion and strength.

Your words matter

You are the narrator of their story.

As a lawyer, I always knew that language mattered. But it wasn't until I became a mother that I realized just how much we, as humans, internalize the language used around us. It can even define us on a subconscious level.

Your words matter in all relationships but to a growing, forming brain, they mean everything.

Around this time, my son didn't like being held by others. Even with friends or family, he'd lean away, burying his head into my shoulder. People would often say, "Oh, he's just shy," and it would make my heart ache. He's not shy. He just loves his mother more than a stranger. He's not hiding; he's seeking comfort in the arms of the one person who has been his whole world from the start. That label, "shy," is limiting and doesn't tell the full story.

Your words not only write the story for your baby, but they also set the stage for the way others view them. You are the narrator, Mama. Be mindful of the story told. Choose wisely and set the example for others to follow.

(A PRAYER FOR TODAY)

God, help me use the gift of speech to narrate my child's world with kindness, love, and patience. May I listen to the inner wisdom and have the confidence to use my voice to advocate for my child when people around them use words that don't sit right with me.

No stage of motherhood is forever—and that is both a relief and a heartbreak

Once I had my baby, I understood the story of Peter Pan a little better. This idea of a place that you could escape to and never get old resonated once I began packing the box of zero to twelve-month clothes in the attic.

My baby was so sweet, so small, and such a miracle, I never wanted him to grow up.

But was I ready for more sleep? Yes.

Was I excited to see him start crawling, take his first step, dance? Of course.

Did I love breastfeeding? Yes.

But was I excited to have my body back and not be constantly concerned whether there was broccoli or cauliflower in the things I was eating? Absolutely.

Each stage in motherhood has parts that make you want to freeze time and parts that you are ready to wash away. That is the beauty in it, and that is what makes our hearts break.

So, enjoy wherever you are today.

(A PRAYER FOR TODAY)

May I embrace today and be settled in my heart so when the time comes to move on to the next chapter, I will feel at peace and move with ease.

Sometimes in the waves of change, our true direction lies below the surface

We uncover the answers to a lot of our decisions and problems when we sit and listen to our inner wisdom. But stillness in motherhood can feel like an impossible luxury. One thing that has always given me comfort is knowing that it's not the length of time that you sit in stillness that matters. Rather, it's that you find it, in whatever form, at any point in the day.

Think of it like a drop of blue food coloring in a glass of water. Sure, more drops will make the water a deeper blue, but even one drop changes the hue and the chemical makeup of the entire glass.

Sometimes one drop is all we need to find the clarity we seek. Other situations and decisions require multiple drops because the stakes are higher.

(A PRAYER FOR TODAY)

God, send your pings to guide me in the right direction loud and clear so that when I quiet the noise of the outside world, the answer is felt acutely within me. May I have the strength to move forward with the decision that reveals itself in these quiet moments.

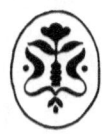

Sip of Self-Care:

The Sit of Determination

The next time you have a decision in front of you, instead of letting it cycle in your mind as you go about your day, set aside five minutes to close your eyes and really *sit* with it. Notice where you feel this decision in your body as you envision the various paths that may unfold depending on the choices you make. Allow the somatic responses in your body to help you select the way forward.

The nine magical minutes

Did you know that not all minutes are created equally? According to Dr. Jaak Panksepp[15], the father of affective neuroscience, there are nine key minutes that hold the most weight for the connection between a parent and child.

They are:

The first three minutes in the morning, right after your baby wakes up.

The three minutes after they come home from daycare or are reunited with you after being away from you for any length of time.

The last three minutes of the day before your baby is put into bed.

It's not to say that the other minutes don't matter, but these are three crucial points in the day that are ripe for connection. Making eye contact, singing to your baby, or holding them during these windows will have an outsized effect on their emotional well-being because they are particularly sensitive times for a child (waking up, returning home, going to bed).

See how you feel when paying attention to these three key transitional times in your baby's day.

Do you notice a difference?

(A PRAYER FOR TODAY)

God, help me to have many genuine moments of heartfelt connection with my baby today. May my baby feel loved, seen, and supported through my words and actions.

Your evolution is seen in the moments you least expect it

How do you know you're changing and evolving?

Unfortunately, (or fortunately), there is no "inner growth" tracker on your Apple watch.

One of my favorite videos to watch is a time-lapse of thousands of pictures of a flower blooming. It lasts three minutes but is comprised of 39,000 individual pictures to detail the flower's growth, moment by moment.

Today, right now, this day, this hour, this minute is like one of those photos, seemingly at a static state, but in reality, in constant motion.

And there will be signs of your evolution, if you look for them.

Look for the confidence that you feel in taking your baby out for a solo stroll (and getting the stroller out of the car) or picking out their favorite foods.

Look for the giggle you and your spouse or partner share when something breaks instead of reacting with frustration.

Look for the gentle response to a restless baby.

Look for the sense of peace when you are up for the eighth time rocking your baby back to sleep tonight.

You are evolving, little by little.

Piece by piece.

(A PRAYER FOR TODAY)

God, help me see signs of my growth in places and spaces I may ordinarily miss. Fill me with gratitude for the changes that are taking place within and around me. Thank you for your guiding hand.

What's that you say?

Of the many jobs you have as a mother, there is perhaps none more important than the Great Interpreter. And the more you become infinitely familiar with your baby's cues, the more you become one of the only people who can decipher what they want.

I speak my son's language in a way no one else can. Two half words, a grunt, and point = he wants the wooden train and banana. I get it.

In a way, you become your baby's translator, speaking the unspoken with a kind of intuitive fluency. It's one of your superpowers, but it can also feel like a lot of pressure because when the language is still known only by you and your baby, it can make it challenging for your partner or community of caretakers to step in and help.

But remember, the more you involve others—your partner, family, friends— the more fluent they'll become in your baby's language. It's not about perfection, it's about practice.

And knowing that your baby can communicate and be heard by others will give you the peace of mind to take the time you need for your own self-care and mental health. It doesn't all have to fall on you, but you do have to be willing to allow others in.

No one will ever do it quite like you, but you giving them the chance to try makes the journey a little lighter for everyone.

(A PRAYER FOR TODAY)

May I be open to letting others learn the language of my baby so I can lean on my community for support.

Nurture what nurtures you too

When you become a mother, the calculation shifts. You are no longer the center of your own universe. Where your life used to focus on your own schedule, needs, and wants, those have now taken a back seat and have maybe even been moved to the trunk. Even so, many mothers (me included) have wondered at some point throughout these past eleven months whether something they did was selfish. I recently went out for a dinner that went later than expected and toward the end of the evening, I could barely enjoy myself because I was worried my baby needed me.

The truth is that being a parent means being tested in every single "selfish" area of our life: we eat second, shower when we can, fit in bits of self-care around our baby's schedule, even hold our pee from time to time when we are "nap trapped" (because who wants to wake a sleeping baby? Not me!). And, of course, there are times when it is biologically necessary to put your baby's needs ahead of your own, but somewhere along the line, it no longer becomes necessary *every time*, it just has become a practice, a habit that is just muscle memory. It feels good to provide, to care, to be needed, but if we constantly dim our light, allocate energy for everyone and everything except ourselves, and move our needs further down the line, it can lead to resentment and/or isolation.

So today, I invite you to start bringing your needs and wants to the forefront once again. It's about striking the right balance of using your time, energy, and resources to take care of not just your baby, but you as well.

(A PRAYER FOR TODAY)

God, remind me often that I am also worthy of love and give me peace that in doing things for myself, I become a better mother.

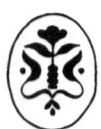

Sip of Self-Care:

Take yourself on a date this week. It doesn't have to be multiple hours, it can be a fifteen-minute trip to the coffee shop where you buy a pastry, find a table alone, and sip your favorite beverage. Feel what it is like to exist in your own energetic field. Use this as a time to refuel and recharge, knowing that in doing so, you are raising your vibrations in every capacity. We send ourselves a subconscious message of empowerment when we give back to ourselves in this way.

Friendship in bloom

A fascinating study from Yale University and the University of California[16] found that the chemistry drawing friends together might originate from shared DNA. The study found that friends tend to be more genetically similar to each other than to strangers, about as closely related as fourth cousins (or about a 1 percent overlap of genes)! This subtle genetic connection might help explain the deep, almost instinctual bonds we form with certain people, making our friendships feel more destined than accidental. For new mothers, this finding has meaningful implications. Navigating matrescence can be more manageable with a strong network. And if your greater family unit doesn't live in proximity or is particularly challenging, the village of women around you becomes even more vital.

Scientists call this "functional kinship," but I like to think of this as bees tending to flowers. The bees are naturally drawn to certain plant species, cultivating their mutual growth and vitality just as we are instinctively drawn to friends for reasons beyond our conscious understanding. These friendships don't need to look a certain way, but they do need to *feel* a certain way. They should *feel* rich in love and empathy, supportive and nurturing.

In the women I interviewed for this book, I asked this question: "If you could have more of something in the first year of motherhood, what would it be?" The answer, time and time again, was community.

Just as pollination is essential for the health and propagation of plants, nurturing our female friendships, finding the right flowers, can lead to deep enduring bonds that support our well-being and happiness.

So, notice who you feel drawn to. Get outside your comfort zone. Whether it's intentionally utilizing the power of social media or online support groups, or even attending a Mommy and Me yoga class in your area, begin making little deposits in your social network so you can bloom together.

(A PRAYER FOR TODAY)

God, send me the women in my life who are meant for me as we witness, hold, support, and nurture one another. Guide my intuition to recognize budding kinships and give me the confidence to step out in faith to feed those friendships that nourish my soul.

Your sacred task

Your sacred task as a mother is to be a witness to your baby and reflect a sense of belonging back to them. We all long to be seen by the ones we love, but a child longs deeply to be fully seen by their parents, and especially their mother.

Early on, my partner encouraged our son to say "Dada" over and over. Endlessly, in fact. And as it turns out, his first word was . . . you guessed it—Dada!

I was initially a bit disheartened, but I recently heard of a theory for why this is that made me smile: Many babies say "Daddy" first because they don't see themselves as separate from their mothers. There would be no reason to call out for her as she's a part of them. She's always there, and they are seamlessly intertwined.

And it reminded me that I don't have to *do* anything to be a good mother. I just have to be my true self, reflecting back the goodness and love my baby has within them. How freeing. I *get to* simply listen and witness, protect them when needed, and encourage their wingspan expansion when the time is right.

These ways of mothering send the message that simply says *I am so happy you're here with me,* which on a subconscious level confirms how valuable our children are and how much their presence and voice are wanted.

This is the heart of motherhood. This is our sacred task.

(A PRAYER FOR TODAY)

May I recognize my innate worthiness and capableness as a mother. May I continually reflect the love within my child back to them so they may stand tall in their self-worth.

The space between

Have you ever felt the feeling of "I've arrived"?

I'm not sure I have, or if I have, it's been short-lived. When I reflect, much of my time is spent in pursuit. Do you ever feel this too? That the moments of simply *being* seem to slip away, overshadowed by the pursuit of what's ahead?

The truth is that most of our life exists in the in-between moments.

Especially in motherhood, there are very few destinations you can sit in long enough to celebrate before you are "on the road again," in route to the next.

And when we focus on always getting "there," we forget that our "here" right now is actually the "there" that our sights were set on from before.

I like to think of the in-between moments as the pauses in a song, where the silence or unspoken melody is as meaningful as the lyrics themselves in shaping the rhythm and depth of the music.

So, I invite you to embrace the in-between moments, savor them even. Because they are the threads that weave together the fabric of our lives, connecting one moment to the next with subtle beauty and significance.

(A PRAYER FOR TODAY)

God, help me reorient my gaze from the horizon and instead focus on the direction of my footsteps I'm taking right here and now, one foot in front of the other. May I recognize the importance of savoring the space between where I am and where I am headed.

Everyday transcendence

A woman at the airport today commented on what a "happy baby" I have. I looked down at my little guy, and he smiled BIG back at me. I returned the smile and giggled to myself. That smile has become everything to me. It can turn my whole day around. Sometimes we get so caught up in the day-to-day, the decision-heavy routine of motherhood, that we forget to stop and marvel at the ordinary moments that have been transformed into the extraordinary.

And this is the meaning of transcendence—seeing the extraordinary in the ordinary. How lucky are we that some of the things that happen every single day in our world, like our baby smiling, are a truly extraordinary occurrence. I know you've felt it when seeing your baby's whole face light up.

This is transcendence—seeing beyond the trees to the light peeking through the clouds. How can we find more of these sacred pauses to witness and marvel at throughout the day, capturing the essence of the moment within our heart span? How beautiful and blessed is this life we are living. And the good news is, the more we look for it, the more we find it.

(A PRAYER FOR TODAY)

God, reveal the sacredness of each moment in my life. May I be awestruck at the beauty sprinkled throughout my day.

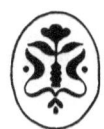

Sip of Self-Care:

Start a mini journal. You can keep it in the Notes app in your phone or in a miniature journal in your purse. When a moment happens with your baby or you feel empowered as a woman, mother, partner—anything that lights you up—jot down a few words in your journal. It is meant to be quick, but when you look back, I promise you will be so happy you have this list to recall those little phrases and experiences that add up to the heartbeat of your mothering journey.

You are interconnected

As a mildly rebellious teenager, I was convinced my mother had a tracker on me. There would be times when my best friend and I would be sneaking out of her window when we'd suddenly see the headlights of my mom's car driving around the block of my friend's house—at 1:30 a.m.! She didn't always catch me, but in the morning she would say things like "Is everything all right? I had a weird feeling that something wasn't right last night." She always knew. It was uncanny. Her instincts were strong.

Now that I'm a mother, I know my maternal instinct is growing every day too. My baby and I are forever connected. Motherhood creates an immeasurable bond of love, connection, and protection you feel toward your baby. You are hardwired to feel the way you do for that sweet soul you ushered earthside. You can anticipate their needs, even when the decisions feel overwhelming, and intuitively care for them and provide them with the type of nourishment they need.

So, the next time the feeling of "not enoughness" runs through your mind, remind yourself of this fact: Your baby is a part of you, and you are forever connected, Mama. No matter how old they are. No matter where they are. No matter what.

(A PRAYER FOR TODAY)

Dear God, thank you for the beautiful and intuitive connection you've created within my baby and me so that we are forever attuned to each other.

Embrace the pace

Now that your little one is crawling, possibly walking, or just moving more generally, you may notice their sense of independence as they test their own capability for doing things on their own. This growth spurt is beautiful, but at times, it also slows us down. The point is that it's meant to. Let it.

Around this time, my son started really hating the stroller and the carrier (unless he was tired). He wiggled and signaled he wanted to get out over and over. Most times we obliged, but then we only made it halfway around the block, which was frustrating when we intended to do a much longer walk. One day, however, we ended up talking to a few of our neighbors around the corner from our house because we were walking so slowly. We made small talk, relishing in the company of new friends, and for the next few years of living there, we regularly kept in touch with the people we met that day.

In essence, we fostered relationships we never would have had we kept on our normal pace. The simple truth is that our babies do slow us down, but if we embrace the pace in which they operate, we may find a whole new world that comes into focus.

(A PRAYER FOR TODAY)

God, help me slow down to enjoy the people and experiences you put in my path. Open my eyes to the moments that will blur if I pass by them too quickly.

God can use you as you exist today

For most of my life I played the "I'll be happy when . . ." game.

I thought once I graduated from college, once I finished law school, once I got my first job, once I met my soulmate, then I would slow down and be truly content. Once I had all these things in order, only then could I start to help others or live my purpose. But I was wrong. I could have started at any moment.

Looking back, I see that God was always waiting, ready to step in as soon as I was open to making a difference. Some of my greatest moments have happened when I thought my life was a mess. I worked on high treason trials in Namibia in law school when I was going through a deep reckoning with who I wanted to be. I opened a meditation studio in Los Angeles when I was at the height of a new travel schedule for my law job. I had a baby during COVID. I don't believe that you have to tough it out or "do it all," but I did learn to embrace where I was instead of waiting for the conditions to be perfect.

And here is what I know now to be true: We don't have to be perfect to create incredible ripples in the lives of others. We don't have to have a lot in order to give. We don't have to know everything to teach others.

We just have to open ourselves to the possibilities of the plans God has set out for us.

(A PRAYER FOR TODAY)

God, reveal yourself and your plan in the moments I feel hopeless and lost. Remind me that I am always in transition but that I am still the product of your creation, and that is a remarkable thing. I am meant to be exactly where I am on my way to where I am going.

Our input guides the output

I invite you to unclench your grip on what motherhood looks like and see what it could be, without force, without control, and without needing it to look a certain way. When we are so set on the outcome in a given situation, there's no room for possibility, for the unexpected, for the beautiful parts we could have never fathomed in our wildest dreams. When we are set on the outcomes, we are attached to predictability, trying to follow a path that has already been taken by others. When we seek to control every aspect of our lives, our expectations become the focus, which almost always leads to disappointment, stress, and anxiety because we can't see the twists and turns like God can.

Instead, ask yourself how you are pouring into yourself. How are you feeding your soul? Essentially, what are your inputs? *That* is within your control, so it's a good place to start.

(A PRAYER FOR TODAY)

God, help me feed my soul with the ingredients to feel a sense of wholeness and fulfillment. May my eyes be opened to what I am feeding into my soul. May I surrender to what the final product looks like in the end. You see the bigger picture; make it a delicious life.

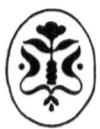

Sip of Self-Care:

Let's look at where to focus your input. Close your eyes and take three breaths. As you do, notice where in the body you feel tension or tightness. Then ask yourself these questions:

- What is causing this tension? Is it emotional, energetic, or physical tension I am holding here?

- How can I relieve this pain or discomfort?

- How can I prevent this pain or discomfort from creeping back up in the future?

There will be a "last" for everything

Navigating sleep for our baby was always hard for us, and it may be for you as well. Crib, bed-sharing, bottle or breastfeeding—no matter what path you have chosen, I want to remind you that there will be a "last" for everything.

A last time they want to be held.

A last time they wake up multiple times per night.

A last time they want their pacifier.

A last time they nurse.

A last time they take multiple naps.

A last time they call out for you in the night.

This is not to say you should give into their every request for fear of never getting the moment again. My point is that it is a relatively short window of time so don't be hard on yourself if you have chosen what feels like the unsustainable option. It doesn't have to be sustainable because your baby will be changing and heading into the next phase soon enough. When we grapple with the impermanence of it all, it becomes a little easier to sit in the hard, in the messy. One day, you might even wish those "lasts" hadn't come so quickly.

(A PRAYER FOR TODAY)

Give my heart contentment and endurance to withstand the hard moments, knowing that they, too, will soon pass. Guide me back to gratitude again and again for the bright light that my baby is in my world.

The potent medicine of prayer

I wrote the prayer below in my journal today. I then said it aloud with my son once in the morning, once before each of his naps, and once again right as he was going down to bed for the night. By the end of the day, I felt that it was written not just on the paper but also on the hearts of my baby and me.

Writing down our prayers and speaking them into existence is a love letter to God. And even more beautiful, it's a response to God's love letter to us, delivered through the blessings we are given and the beauty that surrounds us. It doesn't have to be long. A ten-second prayer will do, but it's speaking to God regularly, as you would in any relationship, that makes your spiritual connection stronger.

Simple, but true, prayer is more potent than any other medicine.

(A PRAYER FOR TODAY)

Dear God,

Thank you for this life,

For the oceans that roar,

For the sun that shines,

For the birds that keep us looking up,

And for all the people,

you have planted by my side.

Motherhood opens the door for a personal and spiritual revolution

In the early *days* after birth, people always ask you how you're doing. In the early *months* of postpartum, people check in to see how the transition is going and how much sleep you are getting. Eventually, though, the questions and check-ins seem to dry up because society has deemed postpartum to be only a few months—six tops, but no more than that.

The truth is that the postpartum period, the true birthing of the mother, can take years. Nikki McCahon, Matrescence Educator, points out that whereas the birth of a baby can be defined by a singular moment in time, the birth of a mother is a far more complex process. It's an unfolding, a true becoming.

And some say that the becoming never really ends. This makes sense to me. The same way that your transition from adolescence to adulthood is permanent, the transition into motherhood, into matrescence, is a lifelong process. I feel that deeply these days, as I am sure you do too. What an opportunity for reinvention, to bloom in ways you have always wanted to.

A woman lives many lives within her one lifetime with each pregnancy and birth and postpartum period. This life you are living today is sacred. It's gritty at times, and it's nuanced always. But I believe motherhood is the biggest revolution you will ever take part in. Allow yourself to step into your insurgence and reimagine the world you want for yourself and your baby.

The best revolutions are led in love. And you, Mama, have no shortage of that.

(A PRAYER FOR TODAY)

God, give me the courage to continue revolutionizing my path as a mother. Thank you for every evolution I am stepping into.

Motherhood is an act of radical optimism

Motherhood is a sacred rebellion, a powerful embrace of what is possible when we break free from the limiting beliefs and patterns we've inherited. It is a rebellion against the dysfunctional childhoods (or parts thereof) we've witnessed. It's a loving declaration that things will be different this time.

And taking a stand for yourself, breaking away from old familial thought patterns, intergenerational behaviors, and traits that have caused more harm than good is an act of sheer bravery. For you are not only healing your own heart but also lifting the entire lineage that has come before you. The strength of your motherhood will surpass what you've known, because the foundation your parents built is now the floor from which you rise.

This is your chance to create something brand new, to build it better than it was, and to make it your own by creating new traditions, new ways of nurturing, and new bonds that reflect the love and wisdom you've always had deep in your soul. So, forge forward. It takes a lot, but the beauty of the transformation is so worth the journey.

(A PRAYER FOR TODAY)

God, give me the strength to continue showing up bravely for myself, my baby, and the family and life I am building for us. It is safe to break away from old ways of being, doing, and connecting. It is safe to release the behaviors and traditions that caused grief, sadness, shame, pain, and other wounding. It is safe to release it all with love and be who you call me to be—an emissary of love, light, and compassion.

Sip of Self-Care:

Breathwork and the Gates of Transformation

When negative thoughts spiral, your breath can help you shift and reset. In breathwork, each breath has three "gates"—the inhale, the pause, and the exhale. These gates act as thresholds for transformation, offering a chance to realign.

Start with a deep inhale, the first gate, inviting courage and intention. Pause for five seconds at the second gate, the stillness where negativity begins to loosen its hold. Then, release with a slow, steady exhale, the third gate, carrying away what no longer serves you.

This simple rhythm—inhale, pause, exhale—disrupts negativity and grounds you in clarity. Whenever you feel overwhelmed, return to the gates of your breath and trust their power to guide you back to balance.

Life is a series of tiny miracles, if only we can notice them

As I washed the dishes tonight, I noticed the warm water dripping over my hands. At that moment, I looked up to see my little one falling asleep in the swing while my favorite Vance Joy song seeped over the living room speakers.

In that space, suspended between the ordinary and the sacred, I realized how much beauty there is in these small moments. It made me realize that life, like a mosaic, is made up of countless little pieces. Sometimes we just see the small dots, but when we take a step back, we notice that those tiny imprints of moments make up the picture of our lives.

The beginning of all creations begins with a tiny stroke. And then another one. And another one. The masterpiece is made not by one grand gesture but by the accumulation of tiny, beautiful acts that we sometimes don't even notice at the time. Each dish washed, each song played, each peaceful breath taken, is a part of something far more profound than we might realize in the rush of life.

(A PRAYER FOR TODAY)

God, let me find joy in the small things, the everyday moments, the in-betweens. Because that is where your love resides most.

The irony is that acceptance is a prerequisite to change

Today, I ask you to sit with acceptance; it's one of the hardest things for us as mothers to come to terms with, and here's why: We have to accept (and acknowledge) what *is* before we can muster the energy to change it.

Self-acceptance takes us from powerlessness to powering *through*. Despite our circumstances.

By accepting it all—the hard, the ugly, the sweet, the calm, the chaos—we come to a steady state long enough to see clearly where and what we want to change. It doesn't mean quitting, giving up, or waving your proverbial white flag. It means giving yourself and your baby and those around you extended grace, compassion, and love. It means witnessing people for who they are, who they choose to be. It means being willing to stay open to the possibilities while coming to a deeper understanding of witnessing the present moment instead of bypassing it or wishing for the future to be here already.

It means loving yourself, accepting yourself wholly as you are right now, and who you've been, so you can step into who God calls you to be as a mother.

When you can extend this grace and acceptance to yourself first, then extend it to your baby and those around you, it will become easier. The muscle memory starts to form, and it leads to a life well lived and a life well loved.

(A PRAYER FOR TODAY)

God, teach me how to lean into gracious acceptance, love, and compassion—toward myself and others around me.

Faith as your cornerstone

A cornerstone refers to the first stone set in the construction of a masonry foundation, and it is of vital importance since all other stones are set in reference to this stone, thus determining the position of the entire structure. In our lives, a cornerstone is something that is essential, indispensable, or foundational to us. It represents a crucial element upon which everything else depends.

What serves as the building blocks on which you are building your life and your baby's? What if it was faith (trust)? How would that change your posture? Your confidence to stand up tall, knowing that it will all work out?

Faith in your ability as a mother. Faith in your beautiful baby. Faith in the family you are growing and expanding. Faith in your journey. Faith in who God is calling you to be. Faith in your relationships. Faith in your career/ business journey. It doesn't mean you don't have an awareness of reality, it simply means that no matter what, your faith is the foundation of your strength.

Some cultivate their faith through prayer and worship, others through meditation and reflection, and others through art, music, writing, or physical movement.

Whatever your faith practice is, lean into it and deepen it. Make it your cornerstone.

(A PRAYER FOR TODAY)

Guide me to walk deeper in faith so that I am thoroughly nourished, rooted, and grounded.

Let your dreams create vivid visions for your life

Dreams are a remarkable testament to the power of the human brain. As a Pisces, I have always had my head in the clouds to some degree, tapping into the imagination and creativity deep within me. But since becoming a mother, I have wondered whether some of the dreams I once had were stale, or still alive, and in some cases, whether they were still possible.

I see you, Mama. You have a heart full of dreams, new ones perhaps from the ones you might have had before motherhood. Perhaps ones that now involve you and your baby and family. And then some dreams just for you.

Each dream is a whisper of what could be—not a rigid plan, but the seeds of a vision that invites us to imagine, feel, and gently shape the future with our heart's desires. In this space, dreams dance in harmony with our deepest yearnings, guiding us with an ever present, nurturing light.

Unfolding like a delicate design of possibility and hope. Unlike the assertive, goal-driven nature of masculine ambition, dreams embrace a gentle feminine energy within them. They flow with a grace that allows for exploration and intuition, if only we let them.

Let your thoughts run wild for your dreams. You haven't lost your fire, your soul, your essence. You've deepened it. You're stepping into the essence of matriarch, wise woman, and a realignment of who you are. This is your time to start as you mean to continue. To chart a new course for your lineage. To rewrite old stories and transform into the wildest, most liberated version of yourself that motherhood is gracing you with the opportunity to be.

(A PRAYER FOR TODAY)

My dreams are good for me, for my baby, and for all of us. These big dreams of mine, I'm going to let them shine.

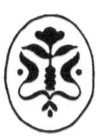

Sip of Self-Care:

Dreaming in the Quiet

Tonight, light a candle and sit in stillness for a few moments. Close your eyes and breathe deeply, letting the flame remind you of the fire within.

Bring to mind one dream that feels alive for you right now. It might be personal, family-centered, or a wild vision for the future. Hold it gently in your heart without trying to shape it—just feel its presence.

Whisper to yourself: "This dream is good for me. This dream is possible."

Let the simplicity of this ritual honor the power of your dreams, reminding you that they are not just wishes but seeds of transformation waiting to bloom.

Self-love as an exploration

Self-love is typically talked about in terms of the things we do for ourselves like getting a massage, having our hair or nails done, meditating, reading, etc. But self-love is not a destination or an accomplishment, it's an exploration of what feels good in your body and headspace.

True self-love is a quiet, gentle listening to the rhythm of your own being. When we tune in, we connect to the part of us that remembers we are nature. Like flowers waiting for the rain, there are parts of us longing to be nourished. This is a powerful energy to call forward—to love yourself fully. It is something we are born with but that we lose along the way. Your baby may be smiling at themselves in the mirror or enamored with their hands—that's it. That is self-love.

Sure, nail appointments and long baths are great, but it's not the activity that is the loving part, it's the time you have carved out to explore your inner waters, the depths of your heart space.

(A PRAYER FOR TODAY)

May I carve out space and time to really get to know myself, and may I shower myself with the same tenderness I give to others.

Remember your Roman Empire

Don't worry, I am not about to dive into a history lesson (although that is one of my favorite subjects). The phrase "someone's Roman Empire" can be used metaphorically to refer to something that is very important, influential, or central to a person's life or identity. It suggests something that holds significant power or influence in their world, much like the Roman Empire did in ancient history.

Generally speaking, my Roman Empire is motherhood. And I am sure yours is too. But let's get more granular. What about your experience holds immense importance and influence in your life? Is it creating a loving home that is warm and nurturing? Is it cultivating curiosity by fostering an environment where your baby's inquisitiveness and zest for learning thrives? Is it encouraging and participating in creative projects, from art to music, that bring joy? Is it cherishing the intimate peaceful times spent together, like bedtime stories or quiet walks? Is it celebrating diversity by introducing and immersing your family in different cultures and perspectives to broaden their understanding and empathy? Is it inventing special personalized family rituals that hold deep sentimental value and create lasting memories?

What stuck out to you? Is there something else that comes to mind? You may have been nodding your head to a few of these, and that's okay. It's not about choosing *one* per se. Instead, it's about finding clarity on the elements that hold value to you as these will help shape your daily actions and sense of purpose.

(A PRAYER FOR TODAY)

God, help me discover my Roman Empire, the heart of my purpose as a mother. May I remember that it will be different for everyone and that I am equipped with my own recipe for motherhood that will satiate and nourish my child. Guide me to find and nurture what is most precious to me and my family in this sacred role.

You are the molder

Recently, in a yoga class, we explored the profound ways in which we shape our own lives. But what is truly miraculous about motherhood is that we extend this power beyond ourselves to mold the lives of our entire household. Women have been chosen by God to be the very seed of creation, the sacred vessels through which life flows and unfolds.

You are the architect of space and time, sculpting not just your own journey but also influencing the emotional, intellectual, and spiritual development of your child. In doing so, you help shape the humanity of tomorrow, nurturing the future generation while also healing and transforming the legacy of the past—our ancestors' stories and struggles.

In essence, the spirit of a woman is the foundation of society itself. Let this knowledge be your guiding force, especially in moments when you feel weak, helpless, or overwhelmed. Within you lies immense power. You are the antithesis of those feelings—possessing immense power within your voice, your heart, and your hands.

You are the molder, Mama, shaping not only your own destiny but also the world around you.

(A PRAYER FOR TODAY)

God, thank you for trusting me to guide my baby and my household. May I hear your whispers at every twist and turn. May I always feel the confidence that you have in me and stand tall because of it.

Faith over fear

What is the opposite of trust? Fear. In motherhood, fear can be overwhelming, its volume cranked up to an unbearable level. The problem with fear is that it consumes precious energy, spiraling through our minds. But it doesn't stop there; fear can easily settle into the body, where it lingers, holding us captive.

One powerful example of this is in the hormone prolactin. In the first few months after giving birth, prolactin floods a mother's body. It's the hormone responsible for milk production and is often referred to as the "mothering hormone" because it strengthens the bond between mother and child. Interestingly, though, prolactin also helps to calm aggressive behavior in mothers, to instead direct that energy to care and nurture their baby.

In this way, while it is instinctual to protect, we also need to be mindful of not letting fear take over. Fear often comes from the feeling of losing control, but the truth is, Mama, that you can navigate anything. If fear is generated in the mind, trust can be generated there too. I invite you to start using this formula whenever fear creeps in. In moments of fear, remember the acronym STIR to help guide you back to trust and intuition:

> S—Stop and acknowledge the fear. What is it trying to teach you? What's the source?

> T—Trust that you are capable. Let go and surrender the fear to a higher power. Allow things to unfold in a way you might not have expected.

> I—Intuition.: Trust your body. It's your wise guide. Let your inner knowing lead you to the right path.

> R—Reframe: Turn the fear into a gift. What can you learn from this moment? How can it strengthen you?

In moments of fear, STIR and reconnect to your strength, trust, and intuition. You have everything you need within you.

(A PRAYER FOR TODAY)

God, help me choose faith over fear, trust over fear, and my inner knowing over fear. Lead me where my feet could never wander without it.

Sip of Self-Care:

Scented Serenity Meditation

Light incense somewhere you can see it clearly. Sit in a comfortable position and take a deep, whole-body breath, allowing the sweet scent of the incense to fill your lungs. As you exhale, imagine releasing any tension or worries. Now, focus on the delicate dance of the incense smoke. Watch as it rises gracefully, swirling and twirling in intricate patterns. As you meditate on the swirling tendrils of incense, allow yourself to settle into the sweet state of surrender.

Create the adventure of your mothership

Sometimes it's just easier to follow the directions on the GPS (that's my take, unfortunately, not my husband's). Other times, no matter how many routes the GPS shows you, you are met with detours, diversions, and road closures. As frustrating as this may feel, sometimes the road less traveled is the one we need to experience. It's in those moments that we turn inward and rely on our inner compass and sense of direction (values) to guide us toward the next turn, to arrive at our destination with ease and excitement (and potentially, on time).

Motherhood is a lot like this. It's mapped out with an end destination and the best intentions. Yet the journey is full of unexpected twists and turns. The best part? You get to choose and create your own adventure. You get to set the schedule that fits with your rhythm. You set the guidelines and create the motherhood manual that works for you—building it as you go. You decide what you will and won't do when you receive feedback and guidance from others (the GPS). You have the power to curate your village, whether or not it aligns with the one you were born into or the support you thought you'd receive. You get to rise after birth in ways that nourish your soul, not according to society's expectations. You get to redefine who you are and what kind of mother you want to be.

In short, you're the captain of your mothership. You choose the destination, and when life asks you to take a detour, you look for the glimmers of light and hope, trusting the journey is leading you exactly where you need to be.

(A PRAYER FOR TODAY)

Dear God, give me the grace and wisdom to continue trusting the direction you are guiding me toward, especially when I don't quite understand it yet. Guide my vision, my direction. May I courageously set foot into the unknown, knowing that I am held in the palm of your hand.

Cultivate a curious mindset

I was in a yoga class today and the teacher invited us to imagine our body and mind as one big house with many levels and hidden rooms—a mansion of sorts, if you will.

She said that it was our option whether to go into each of the rooms of the house or to leave the doors shut. It was our decision to turn on the lights or keep it dark. It was our prerogative to clean up certain messes or let them be. It was our decision to answer the door when the doorbell rang or leave it unanswered. Essentially, we could choose to be curious or not.

Although we have one body and one mind, we are layered creatures. The more we can walk around the "house" and get to know the layout, the more confident we feel about what belongs in there and what needs to go—the more we can start loving the home for all its beauty and flaws.

So, when you notice yourself having a certain feeling, reaction, gut ping, or response of any kind, explore it. What is it there to show you? To teach you?

(A PRAYER FOR TODAY)

God, guide me to approach my life with curiosity and an open heart, seeking answers and wisdom in every experience. Grant me the courage to explore, learn, and grow, finding joy and meaning in the journey of discovery.

Feel your inner light; free your inner vixen

I know some days can be long and some nights, even longer. Weeks turn into months, and time can blend together. In the midst of the transition, the profound initiation, you may not have had a moment to truly *catch your breath*. Take a moment to breathe now. To witness yourself. To see yourself, outside and inside. Not just the mother, but the *whole* you. The woman within. The creative, fun, playful, sassy inner vixen.

The word "vixen" always felt sexualized to me, and I hesitated to really adopt the word when describing myself until I discovered that it means a female fox. As I dove deeper into its origins and usage, I uncovered that it is a word used to describe a woman with beauty that is subtle yet captivating, her demeanor playful yet dignified. The vixen's ability to thrive in diverse environments reflects a woman's capacity to face challenges with resilience and courage. It's a woman who possesses an inner fire that fuels her journey, making a vixen a symbol of elegance, cunning, and empowerment.

Yes, a vixen is something to *be*.

Just because you are a mother doesn't mean you need to completely let go of your sense of style and self. You can still look sleek, sexy, and well put together *and* be comfortably dressed without breaking the bank or doing a massive closet overhaul. Just because you are a mother doesn't mean you need to put solo time or date nights with your partner or girls' nights in/out aside. Sure, they might not happen every single week or as often as you'd experience it in the past, but I encourage you to still make it a point to stay connected with yourself and others. Just because you are a mother doesn't mean you put yourself last on the checklist.

Let your inner light invite the vixen within to run wild and free. Honor *her*, too.

(A PRAYER FOR TODAY)

On days when it feels like time is at a standstill, guide me to find the lightness in my being, the lightness in each moment, and to cherish myself, my body, my baby, and the people I am blessed with in this life before me.

Gratitude, Grace, and Grit: Your motherhood companions

The 3G's, as I like to call them, will carry you through your journey during the Mother Year and beyond.

Gratitude for all the moments, for the simple privileges and pleasures (that often go unappreciated when we are caught up in our day-to-day), for the support system around us, for our bodies, for our babies, for our partners, and for our village that holds us and shows up for us. As I type these words with one hand, my baby warm on my chest, it's a reminder that simply being here *is* enough.

Grace for all the moments you've felt guilt, shame, anger, resentment, sadness, loneliness, isolation, grief, frustration. For the times you've felt like you're not enough. For the times you've had the urge to burn down a sacred relationship or friendship or lash out. For the times you've simply wanted a moment of space from your baby. It's all part of the journey, and it's totally normal. Give yourself grace.

Grit for all the days when it feels like you're about to lose yourself amid the chaos, for the moments that can be heartbreaking like returning to work or juggling the unwavering requests of this world. For the days, weeks, and months that feel unending in some ways but speedy in others. For the times you feel like you're not cut out for this initiation. For the times you face everything that comes your way, head up, heart led, and faith first.

You are beyond capable, and you are powerful beyond measure. Remember your 3G companions are always on your side because they are within you. *They are you.*

(A PRAYER FOR TODAY)

God, guide me to tap into gratitude, grace, and grit every single moment. May I witness this within myself and extend it as a token of love to others around me.

Sip of Self-Care:

Reflecting on Grit, Grace, and Gratitude

Today, pause for a moment of reflection. Think back over the past week and identify one example of grit—a moment where you persevered through challenge. Recall a moment of grace—where you extended compassion to yourself or someone else. Finally, honor a moment of gratitude—a spark of thankfulness that lifted your spirit.

Let this simple practice remind you of your strength, your kindness, and the blessings that surround you. Each of these moments is a testament to the beauty of your journey.

Awaken your inner knowing

Midwife and human rights advocate Ibu Robin Lim[17] describes the meta meaning of pregnancy, birth, and the motherhood experience as a process to "awaken your inner knowing." It wasn't until I became a mother that I felt I truly understood this.

Motherhood is a profound transformation that touches every part of your being. Giving birth changes you—physically, emotionally, and psychologically. It's a fierce initiation into the parts of yourself you've perhaps ignored or tucked away. Matrescence, the journey of becoming a mother, beckons you to confront these dormant parts, to reconnect with a simpler, more child-like sense of wonder. In the midst of the beautiful chaos and joy, you step off autopilot and begin to rediscover a new way of being. It is an invitation to embrace the simplicity of being present. This journey is not just about nurturing the child in your arms, it's also about nurturing your own inner child. It's a path of inner restoration—learning to lovingly care for yourself as you cultivate a deep, loving relationship with your little one.

For many of us, motherhood beckons us to embrace the parts of us that have felt powerless, or the parts of ourselves that have been dormant with desires still burning. Perhaps this means you start a new blog, or a business, or return to a passion or hobby you loved (and set aside in adulthood). Perhaps it's the need to set stronger boundaries around your time and energy, recognizing that as a mother, you are not only protecting your own well-being but also guarding the sacred space for your child. It might even mean learning to advocate for yourself with a fierce yet gentle strength, just like a mother does.

Whatever your path looks like, let your awakening unfold in the whispers of your heart and the pulls of your soul.

(A PRAYER FOR TODAY)

God, thank you for awakening my inner knowing. May I have the courage in each moment to lean into my intuition and to follow her call.

What would you tell your pre-motherhood self?

As you near the close of this transformative first year as a mother, take a moment to honor the wisdom and insights you've gained. This initiation into motherhood is not just about raising your baby, it's about birthing a new version of yourself.

Looking back on your journey, reflect on these questions:

- What pearls of wisdom would you love to share with your pre-motherhood self?

- What insights have you gained about yourself that you wouldn't have known before motherhood?

- What blessings, beyond your baby, do you celebrate openly now?

- What behaviors and relationships have you chosen to release that you never would have before?

- What things do you no longer tolerate that you would have endured before?

- Where has your emotional, energetic, and mental capacity expanded you?

- Where have you softened? Where have you strengthened? And where have you leaned into deeper surrender?

Motherhood is a beautiful meditation, one that brings you closer to your soul while expanding and freeing you from any self-imposed or societally imposed norms and rules. It invites you to lean into your growth edges.

Today, take a moment to reflect on your journey. Celebrate the woman you were, the woman you are, and the mother you're becoming.

Look how much you've grown—and how far you've come!

(A PRAYER FOR TODAY)

God, give me the wisdom to honor my journey, to honor who I've been, who I am, and who you're calling me to be.

There's a whole world in your hands

There's a whole world of play, creativity, love, peace, wonder, adventure, sensitivity, empathy, sass, feistiness, and art in your hands. There's a whole world full of strength, leadership, power, surrender, softness, and emotions in your hands. And this world is currently being cultivated in your baby, in you, and in the relationships you foster and nurture.

This morning, I was sitting on the floor, zoning out—exhausted, caught up in my own thoughts. My son was in his own world too, fiddling with a plastic cup, tapping it against the floor with his little hands. I wasn't really looking at him, just listening to the rhythm, lost in the mess of my mind. Then, out of nowhere, I felt a small soft hand on my cheek. I turned, and there he was—his eyes wide, his mouth open in a grin, and before I could even react, he kissed me: a big wet kiss right on my face and then laid his head on my chest. We both paused. It wasn't planned, just a moment of pure love. And as quickly as it came, he was back to the cup, focused again like nothing had happened.

But I stayed there, still, grounded in that little moment. It was his way of reminding me that I am loved—that even in the midst of my chaos, I am seen. I am enough.

There's a whole world in your hands, Mama—a world that you are shaping in each moment. Through every thought, every word, every action. You're raising tomorrow's leaders, today. God placed you here in your baby's life because only you can guide them and love them in the way you can do.

(A PRAYER FOR TODAY)

God, guide me and be the voice within as I continue to show up for myself, my baby, and my family. May I lead and love just like you do—unconditionally.

Ground your heart in the frequency of mothering

All energy carries a frequency that can be measured in hertz, from the subtle hum of a thought to the powerful vibrations of our emotions. The highest, purest frequency? Love.

As I looked down at my baby's face while he was feeding today, and he looked back up at me with those big wonder-filled eyes, there was no shortage of that high frequency feeling of love.

When the world feels too heavy, too much, when social media, work, partnerships, friendships, and decisions feel overwhelming, take a moment to look at your baby. Allow your relationship to raise the frequency in which you operate.

Can you imagine what your baby must be thinking while staring up at you? I like to imagine my son's coos saying words of affirmation back to me: "You are loved, Mama," "You are so kind, Mama," "You are a beautiful being, Mama."

No one sees you as clearly or as perfectly as your baby. Ground your heart in the reflection of their eyes. Let their gaze remind you of the beautiful frequency you carry—the frequency of mothering, which is nothing less than love.

(A PRAYER FOR TODAY)

God, may my heart overflow with love, so much so that it pushes out those low vibration feelings.

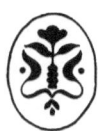

Sip of Self-Care:

Today, when you are looking at your baby and smiling at them, imagine three affirmations they may be sending to your heart space. They may not be able to yet communicate in words, but our babies are operating at that highest frequency of love, especially when they are looking at the person they cherish most in this world—you.

How will you celebrate your birth-day, Mama?

The one-year mark of your journey into matrescence is truly a monumental moment. It's so big that I am intentionally sharing this entry almost two weeks prior to the big day so you can start thinking about how you want to celebrate *you*. Maybe you're planning a grand shindig for your baby, or maybe it will be an intimate gathering with close friends/family. But in addition to honoring your baby's milestone, I want you to pause and think about how you'll celebrate *your* birth-day, Mama. You were reborn the same day as your baby, and that deserves recognition.

For me, I've created a special Rebirth Journal that I will write in only once a year, around this time. In it, I will write a word or phrase that represents the past year—one that encapsulates the highs, the lows, and the transformation. I'll also include a mantra or wish for myself as I move into the next year of motherhood. It's a sacred moment for me to honor the deep journey I've been on and to see the growth over time. Your Mother Year often feels like a lifetime in itself. And once we've made it there, we stand in reverence for the ways in which we have changed. So, celebrate yourself. Because only you know the length to which your soul and heart have been stretched, the profound metamorphosis you've experienced.

Treat yourself to a small cake, or bake one. Light a candle in the quiet of the night or while surrounded by friends. Do something that feels exciting or affirming *for you*.

You are worth celebrating. You are a force, a creation, a rebirth.

(A PRAYER FOR TODAY)

God, as I prepare for my first birth-day in my matrescence journey, I reflect with gratitude on the growth and transformation I've experienced as a mother. Thank you for guiding me through challenges as I cultivate patience and resilience. May I feel the adornment of your love and confidence in my abilities. May I find the energy to celebrate not only my child but also the abundance of love that I am as their mother.

Healing means changing from one state to that of another

Healing is the process of transformation—of shifting from one state to another. After our babies are born, the healing process takes time. And healing requires deep, profound change, which is why this past year may have felt like a whirlwind of physical, mental, and emotional shifts. When you reflect on the word "postpartum," I hope you feel proud of the healing journey you are on because you have been through a great deal, Mama. Birth is one day but postpartum is a lifetime. Don't let anyone tell you otherwise.

Every mother's timeline is unique, but here are just a few of the extraordinary changes your body, mind, and spirit have undergone over the past twelve months:

- *Your brain*: It takes at least four months for brain function and structure to normalize into its postnatal state, reshaping you for deeper connection and care.

- *Your immune system*: It takes six months for your immune system to fully regulate. Certain natural cellular processes that fight off toxins that were suppressed during pregnancy to protect your baby take time to recalibrate.

- *Your body*: It takes six to nine months to regulate the pelvic floor and core muscles to regain balance and strength.

- *Your blood*: It takes at least twelve months for hemoglobin and iron levels to return to normal after the incredible work your body did to sustain life.

- *Your hormones*: It takes up to two years for your hormones to fully stabilize, gently guiding you toward a new equilibrium.

So today, let me remind you that you are healing, even on days when you can't see or feel it. And you are coming out of the other side of this stronger, wiser, and more spiritually connected than before. You are worthy of healing in your own time. You are becoming, in every sense of the word, whole, powerful, and fully you.

(A PRAYER FOR TODAY)

God, heal me in your own time. May I appreciate where I am now and have faith that everything I need will come to me. May I feel protected and supported at this time.

Make the freest human being you know your teacher

Over the past year, you've guided your baby through the wonders of the world, introducing them to shapes, sounds, colors, and flavors. You've taught them words and shown them how to smile, sit up, and walk. From the warmth of the womb to the vast, vibrant adventure of the outside world, you've expanded their horizons every step of the way.

But what about all those lessons you have learned *from* your baby? This uninhibited, untainted, unfiltered little human being is the definition of pure freedom and innocence. We should all strive to live in their image.

Have you noticed how quickly your baby forgives? They don't hold on to grudges within their little bodies and growing minds.

Have you seen how easily they move through the rainbow of emotions? Their expressions are direct and sincere. They don't suppress their experience; instead, they let the emotions of sadness, anger, or frustration flow through and out of their body.

Have you noticed the playfulness that your baby embodies? Everything from a spoon to a crayon is interesting to them. They look at the mundane with a sense of wonder. Can you let this inspire you to release attachment to the outcome of situations or your need to know/have control? For one can only truly play when they are present.

What are some other qualities about your baby that you love?

How can you use those qualities to weave them into the way you show up in your own life?

Class is in session. Let's distill all we can learn from our sweet little teachers.

(A PRAYER FOR TODAY)

Dear God, open my heart and mind to the lessons my child teaches me each day. Help me see through their innocence and curiosity the profound wisdom they bring, guiding me to learn, grow, and love more deeply.

A love note to your little

In this season of summer within your Mother Year, the days may feel long at times, but in hindsight, they swirl by in a dizzying dance that leaves you wanting more and less at the same time.

It's hard to put into words this feeling, but I tried my best as I wrote a love note to my son. I hope it lands softly in your heart space today.

Sometimes I can't remember me before you were here . . .

I'm sure she was driven,

but by different things than I am now.

I'm sure she believed in miracles,

but now I've seen it firsthand as you divinely came into this world.

You have brought out the best parts of me

and you make every day feel like a day to remember,

even in the small moments that would mean nothing to someone else looking in.

You cracked opened my heart and my soul

And the love I have for you is one I'll never be able to fully describe in words.

But I'll spend a lifetime showing you,

showing you what you mean to me.

A lifetime of being your mom

Thank you for making me yours.

(A PRAYER FOR TODAY)

God, thank you for choosing me, out of all the people on this earth, to be the mother to my baby. I now have a better understanding of the love, compassion, and warmth that you feel toward me as your creation.

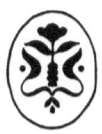

Sip of Self-Care:

A Love Note in Your Voice

Today, take a moment to record a voice note for your baby. It doesn't have to be long or perfectly polished, just let your heart speak. Open the Voice Notes app or your favorite recording app on your phone and let the words flow.

Talk about the love you feel, the milestones you've shared, and the little moments that make your days together so special. Share how proud you are of how far you've both come this year. Your voice will be a precious gift, a keepsake of this season of life.

One day, your baby will hear this recording and feel the depth of your love, not just in the words you say but also in the warmth of your voice. Let this be a simple, heartfelt expression of all that's in your heart right now—a love note carried through time.

The space between effort and ease

When I first became a mother, I believed that the more effort I put in, the better mother I'd be. So, I did as much as I could and was often hard on myself during moments of rest, convinced I should be doing more.

As time went on, my perspective shifted. I began to think that the easier motherhood came to someone, the better she must be at it. So, when things felt hard for me, I saw that as proof of my inadequacies, as though my struggles were a sign I wasn't measuring up. But now I know better.

Motherhood isn't about constant striving, nor is it defined by effortless grace. The truth is, the journey exists somewhere in between—the space between effort and ease. I was kayaking on the lake one starry night and my rhythm felt emblematic of how my mothering had evolved. For a stretch, I paddled steadily, working hard to propel myself forward, gaining momentum. Then I paused, letting up to rest, allowing the kayak to glide effortlessly across the water, savoring the quiet. Occasionally, an unanticipated wave swept me sideways, so I steered to correct my course again. It was this dance—effort followed by rest, action balanced with stillness—that carried me to the other side of the lake. If I hadn't made the effort to turn the paddles, there wouldn't have been movement forward, but if I'd paddled without a break, I would have burned out quickly without having the chance to reach my destination or appreciate how far I had come. Effort and ease. Both are needed.

And that's exactly how motherhood is meant to be.

(A PRAYER FOR TODAY)

Let the moments when motherhood feels easy remind me of what a good mother I am, God, and let me do the same in the moments when it feels like I'm paddling in place.

In the end, love is what lasts

The secret to loving your life? Fill it with love—not just for the big and shiny moments, but for the quiet, everyday ones too. Wake up and embrace this mantra: "It's a privilege to get to be me." This isn't about perfection or arrogance, it's about gratitude. When we focus on what we lack, we betray the beauty that already surrounds us. But when we lean into love and connection, we begin to see the extraordinary within the ordinary.

Start with something as simple and profound as a hug. When you hold your baby, your partner, or a loved one in a warm embrace, oxytocin—often called the "love hormone"—is released. This incredible chemical lowers stress, reduces pain, and deepens the bond between you and the people you hold close.

Let the power of touch remind you of the abundance in your life. Your incredible community. The friends who lift you up. The small but thoughtful ways you spend your time, money, and energy. And your baby? A blessing beyond words, radiating joy into your world.

Your life is overflowing with goodness, Mama. Love it fiercely. Love it fully. Let each hug, each small moment, be a reminder that life is meant to be savored, not rushed through.

(A PRAYER FOR TODAY)

Dear God, help me embrace and love my life exactly as it is now. Grant me gratitude for the blessings, patience for the challenges, and wisdom to find joy and meaning in every experience.

Let us remember the sacredness of our story while we live it

Most people don't like getting older, typically because of the obvious challenges: less flexibility, less energy, less collagen, and more importantly, less time on earth with people they love.

But I'd be willing to bet that if you polled people at the end of their life and asked what period they wanted to relive, most would likely respond that they'd return to the exact chapter you are in now: when the kids are young and there is beautiful chaos swirling around. Where messes pile up, but so do the snuggles. When your baby looks at you like you are all that matters.

So, sit with that for a moment.

You are in such a beautiful chapter even though it has its challenges. This time will be on the highlight reel of your life. You will one day long to rewind your life to relive the moments you are waking up to today.

Why? Because they're raw. Because they're gritty. Because they're humbling. And because they're fleeting.

So, live it fully, Mama. Take it all in. This season may feel challenging, but it's also achingly beautiful.

(A PRAYER FOR TODAY)

God, fill my heart with gratitude for the blessing that is my life. May I feel deeply connected to my baby, my heart, my mind, and my body as I walk in alignment during this season, honoring each moment that is before me.

There are no straight lines in nature

Before becoming a mother, there were parts of my life I would have described as a "straight line." My morning routine was planned perfectly, my days were predictable, and my to-do list was adorned with beautifully inked check marks. But this past year? Nothing has felt straight or linear. It's been full of curves, bends, and circles.

And yet, when I look to the natural world around me, I see no straight lines there either. The organic beauty found in rivers meandering through valleys, tree branches swaying gracefully, rugged mountains rising high—is there anything more beautiful?

These contours symbolize the fluidity of life. So, let the nonlinear journey that has shaped you over the past year be okay. Let it be more than okay. Let it cloak you like the golden light of dawn wraps around the earth.

There are no straight lines in this path of motherhood, only winding roads of learning, growth, and love that shape us as mother and baby.

(A PRAYER FOR TODAY)

God, grant me the wisdom to embrace the curves of life with open arms, trusting in your loving guidance to navigate the twists and turns with grace and resilience. Help me find beauty and growth in every bend, knowing that your plan unfolds in perfect harmony.

Sip of Self-Care:

Part of what makes the "flow" of life feel scary is our fear of the future. How will the path look if it's not straight?

Today, I invite you to try a hand mudra with me. This hand mudra is called the "Lotus" or "Padma Mudra," and it represents the ability to rise above the fear of the unknown, just as the lotus flower floats above the muddy waters on which it sits.

How to practice:

1. First, bring your hands into a prayer pose in front of your heart.

2. Keeping the base of your hands, your thumbs, and your pinkie fingers together, start unfurling your middle, index, and ring fingers. Your hands will resemble a flower blossoming.

3. Close your eyes and take ten to twenty slow, deep breaths. Notice the wave-like, curved sensation of the breath moving through your chest.

When you're ready, open your eyes and surrender to the winding flow of today. Trust that beauty lies in the curves.

The power of perspective

What will really matter a year, or even five years, from now?

That moment when your baby spits up all over themselves and you, especially after you've just had a shower and are finally feeling fresh, clean, and more like yourself . . .

Or when the floor has more baby food than their tummy . . .

Or when your well-meaning family member once again delivers unsolicited parenting advice and you're a step closer to losing your cool . . .

Or that time when all you wanted was a good night's sleep, but you've been awake for hours because your baby is teething or sick . . .

These moments, as difficult as they are in the now, will pass. Time moves on, and what feels heavy today will eventually soften. When we look back a year, or five years, from now, we will likely reminisce about these moments with a sense of bittersweet nostalgia, realizing that they were part of the magic of motherhood—the challenges, yes, but also the tenderness, the rawness, and the growth.

The key to navigating these moments lies in the lens we choose to use. It's all about perspective. When we zoom out, we see that the difficulties are just a small part of a much bigger picture. They are the growing pains, the moments that shape us, that mold us into the mothers we're becoming.

Sometimes a perspective shift is all we need to make it through each day. Zoom out. Reframe. See the whole story, Mama.

(A PRAYER FOR TODAY)

God, give me the grace to accept each moment for what it is. Teach me to have gratitude for the blessings you've given me, for the child you've blessed me with, for the life you are helping me cultivate.

A note on unbecoming

As you approach the one-year mark with your baby earthside, it's natural to reflect on all you've become, on the growth, the milestones, and the transformation of the past year. But today, I invite you to also honor the *unbecoming*.

Matrescence isn't just about expansion, it's also about shedding. It's in the unraveling of old layers, expectations, and stories that you make space for so your truest self can emerge. The unbecoming is just as sacred as the becoming. Over the past year, you've likely let go of many things: habits, identities, and expectations that no longer serve you. Some releases felt gentle; others, like tectonic shifts. These moments of loss are not truly losses, they are but a clearing of space for the woman you are becoming. The process is both quiet and powerful, requiring trust in what's meant to stay and what's meant to go.

As you stand at this threshold, give yourself permission to *exhale*. Step away from what drains your energy, from expectations—yours and others'—that no longer fit. Make space for rest, for nature, for creative expression.

You may feel a deep instinct to protect your energy, a stronger pull toward what truly nourishes you. Honor that feeling. It is guiding you toward what matters most. So, as you reflect on this year, remember: *the unbecoming is just as important as the becoming.* You are not losing anything—you are creating space for the fuller version of yourself to emerge. Rest, release, and allow yourself to unbecome, knowing it is through this process that you will step into the next beautiful chapter of your journey.

(A PRAYER FOR TODAY)

Dear God, during busyness, grant me the precious gift of space to reflect, rest, and be renewed in your loving embrace. Help me find moments of stillness amid the chaos, where I can quiet my mind and listen to the whispers of your wisdom. May these times of solitude be a sanctuary for my soul. Fill me with your peace and rejuvenate my spirit so I may continue to journey with faith and purpose.

You are a miracle, Mama, so live like it

From the dawn of time, countless stars have burned and died, scattering their atoms into the universe. Millions of moments had to align perfectly, ancestors had to survive against unimaginable odds, and life itself had to prevail through every twist of history—for you to be here, in this body, at this exact moment.

Today, I invite you to take a moment and honor yourself for the miracle *you* are.

Honor the life in your bones, the magic in every cell of your body, the power in every fiber of your being. You are not just a person; you are the culmination of stardust and survival, of love and resilience.

You are a work of divine creation, art woven together. The magic and the muse.

That miracle is evident in how you've carried, sustained, and birthed your baby. It shines in the way you lead, the way you nurture and nourish your baby, in the way you show up. Day after day. Time after time.

Can you feel all of life rooting for you? Every atom, every ancestor, every heartbeat of the universe has conspired to bring you here.

You are a miracle, Mama. God made sure of it. Live in that truth.

(A PRAYER FOR TODAY)

Thank you, God, for the miracle that I am, that my baby is, that my life is.

The many thresholds of motherhood

Before becoming a mother, I couldn't envision how it would look. Sure, I'd heard stories and seen glimpses on social media, but the reality for *me* still felt elusive. And yet, here I am, on the other side of that threshold—and now I understand why it's so hard to articulate. Motherhood is an endless well of love yet it challenges you in ways you never expected, pushing you to the edge of your own perceived limitations.

Being a mother has shown me that there is always another threshold. Just when I think I've figured something out, another one appears. And with each new threshold, we must find deeper wells of strength and resilience to keep moving forward—carrying with us the courage to embrace what lies ahead and the faith that we are capable of crossing it.

In many cultures, thresholds are sacred. In Hawaii, for example, it's common to hang wind chimes by the door, symbolizing prosperity and good fortune. The gentle chime of the wind is said to invite positive energy and blessings into the home, marking the transition from one space to the next. It's a reminder that we are always moving forward, and that every doorway we cross offers a new opportunity for growth and transformation.

Arguably, no threshold is more transformative than the one of matrescence. Motherhood teaches us that we are powerful beyond measure while simultaneously inviting us to surrender in ways we never knew possible. As you cross the one-year mark tomorrow, remember how your soul has been transformed in these seasons and how you are on the precipice of a new threshold. Stand tall, Mama. Walk through that door with grace and confidence.

(A PRAYER FOR TODAY)

God, in times of overwhelm, provide me with comfort to ease my worries and the guidance to find my way. Help me see the shimmering glimmers of hope in my baby's eyes and feel your peace amid all this change.

Sip of Self-Care:

Celebrate Your Birth-Day as a Mother

Pause and reflect on where you were one year ago. Picture your life then, and fast-forward through the past twelve months like a mental movie. See the challenges you've faced, the joy you've felt, and the growth you've experienced.

Your brain, body, and intuition have navigated motherhood with incredible strength and resilience. Take a moment to honor this journey and feel gratitude for all you've become.

And here's a reminder: It's your birthday too, Mama. The day your baby was born, a new version of you was born as well. Celebrate yourself by getting your own cake—yes, a separate one just for you. Light the candles, close your eyes, and make a wish for the year ahead. This is a moment to honor your growth, your grace, and the unfolding journey that lies ahead.

The path of motherhood is ever evolving, and you are walking it beautifully. Celebrate that. Celebrate *you*.

Steeping in the initiation that has been your Mother Year

Congratulations, beautiful Mama! You did it! Take a moment to revel in the beautiful, powerful initiation that you've walked through this year . . . as a mother! A whole version of you reborn—stronger, wiser, softer, fiercer, more graceful and compassionate.

This year wasn't easy—it was raw, real, and at times, relentless in its demand for you to grow, stretch, and rise. And yet, here you are. Radiant. Resilient. Rooted in your power. Through the prayers, words, and practices of this book, it's been my deepest privilege to walk alongside you, to remind you that you have never been alone on this journey. Together, we've celebrated your first Mother Year—but here's the beautiful truth: This is only the beginning.

Your growth, your transformation, your deepening understanding of love are the seeds for what lies ahead: the living, breathing, ever-evolving path that is your motherhood. The unfolding doesn't end here, it stretches into a lifetime of Mother Years. Like the wonder years of childhood, your Mother Years will be full of new seasons, thresholds to cross, doors to open, and infinite ways to expand and blossom. Motherhood isn't just one year—it's a lifetime of becoming. With each chapter, the cycle begins again, richer and deeper each time.

Here's to the wonder of your Mother Years.

(A PRAYER FOR TODAY)

Dear God,

Thank You for guiding me through this first year of motherhood. Thank you for the strength I didn't know I had, for the grace that carried me, and for the love that expanded beyond my imagination. As I step forward into the journey ahead, help me to trust the unfolding. Let me meet each new season with an open heart, knowing that you walk beside me through every change. May I continue to grow, to love, and to become the mother you created me to be.

So it ends.

The *first* Mother Year.

And in it's wake, another begins.

We are always evolving.

Always becoming.

Always in process.

Here's to the wonder of

The Mother *Years* ahead.

End Notes

[1] McCahon, Nikki. https://www.nikkimccahon.com/

[2] Ou, Heng, *The First Forty Days: The Essential Art of Nourishing the New Mother* (2016) Harry N. Abrams

[3] Jones, Lucy, *Matrescence: On the Metamorphosis of Pregnancy, Childbirth and Motherhood* (2024) Allen Lane

[4] Douglas J. Blackiston, et al (2008) "Retention of Memory through Metamorphosis: Can a Moth Remember What It Learned As a Caterpillar?" doi: 10.1371/journal.pone.0001736

[5] Taylor-Kabbaz, Amy, *Mama Rising: Discovering the New You Through Motherhood* (2020) Hay House Inc.

[6] Athan, Aurélie. https://www.matrescence.com/

[7] Sacks, Alexandra. https://www.alexandrasacksmd.com/

[8] Blaskey, Zoe, *Motherkind* (2025) HarperCollins

[9] Harrold, Jessie, *Mothershift: Reclaiming Motherhood as a Rite of Passage* (2024) Shambhala

[10] Brené Brown, https://brenebrown.com/art/24339/

[11] ten Boom, Corrie, *The Hiding Place: 35th Anniversary Edition* (2006) Chosen Books

[12] Rohn, Jim. https://www.jimrohn.com/

[13] Dass, Ram. https://www.ramdass.org/

[14] Blaskey, Zoe, *Motherkind* (2025) HarperCollins

[15] Panksepp, Jaak, PhD, *Affective Neuroscience: The Foundations of Human and Animal Emotions* (2004) Oxford University Press

[16] Christakis, N. A., & Fowler, J. H. (2014) "Friendship and Natural Selection." *Proceedings of the National Academy of Sciences* doi:10.1073/pnas.1400825111

[17] Lim, Ibu Robin. https://www.iburobin.com/

Acknowledgments

This book is a labor of love, and I am deeply grateful to those who have supported me along this journey.

To my precious boys, Crusoe and Shiloh, for being the heart of my journey into motherhood. Your presence has inspired every word, every reflection, and every page of this book. You are the reason I write, the reason I grow, and the reason I am continually in awe of the beauty of matrescence.

To my husband, Zac, for walking beside me with patience, love, and understanding. Thank you for letting me write for hours on end, with every spare moment I had for months, and for always supporting my work. Your unwavering belief in me has been my anchor.

To my own mother, Kay, for your endless love, wisdom, and support. You have been my guiding light and a constant source of strength, reminding me of the power of a mother's love.

To God, for planting the seed of this idea in my heart and for guiding me through the challenges and blessings of bringing this book to fruition.

To my mentors, accountability partners, and book doulas, especially Kristina Marie Rose, Kaytlyn Spenner, Laura Thomas, Cat Sager and Erica Galia for your dedication, friendship, and expertise in helping me bring this book to the world.

To the Rooted Beings Mama Circle community, for the endless support, shared wisdom, and connection. Your strength and openness remind me that we are never alone on this path.

To Sabrina Greer, Tania Moraes, and the wonderful team at fEMPOWER, for your guidance, wisdom, and belief in this project.

And finally, to you, the reader. Thank you for inviting *The Mother Year* into your life and for allowing these words to accompany you on your journey into motherhood. I honor you, and I walk beside you in this season of transformation.

With love and gratitude,

Chelsey Scaffidi

(Heartbeat of *The Mother Year*)

Amy Abbott • Jules Acree • Tayler Ansel • Sam Aravopoulos • Heather Barnes • Myriane Elsa Bessette • Christina Blankenburg • Skylar Bodner • Alyssa Brieloff • Tessa Carpenter • Ana Catalina Amador • Kristen Christopher • Brandilyn Clay • Joanna Cohen • Jen Cohen • Holly Curtis • Jade Denberg • Torrey Devitto • Sarah D. Donatelli • Ty Dougherty • Angelika Drake • Onkar Elizabeth Ryan • Andrea Fagenholz • Nev Farah • Sara Flanzraich • Lauren Fleishman • Jordan Friendly • Marika Frumer • Miranda Gale • Erica Galia • Rachel Garahan • Olga Garcia • Alicia Gardner Kennedy • Laura Gilham-Jones • Jacq Gould • Jessica Gross • Natalie Guillermo • Sumner Hanna • Jessica Hargest • Kayleigh Harrigan • Haley Heaton • Sarah Hollingsworth • Erica Ignajatovic • Rachel Jackson • Nicole Jacks • Jaclyn Kaminski-Beneche • Jessie Karlin • Emily King • Mia King Gautreau • Summer Kundo • Akua Lalo • Sherry Landry • Sarah Larson • Misha LaRue • Crystal Lee • Sanetra Longno • Stephanie Margaronis • Liz Mars • Erica Matluck • Adriane McCord • Britta McCrae • McLean McGown • Annalisa McVicker • Nicole Miller • Jen Miller • Abbi Miller • Ellie Montgomerie • Tania Moraes • Elisa Morton • Nicole Moya-Amengual • Kylin Murren • Carson Myers • Nikki Norenberg • Chinny Okpara • Katie Onusic • Roxy Peake • Katie Powell • Carrie Rae • Jenna Reiss • MJ Renshaw • Nikki Riccoboni • Julia Saenz Rosenthal • Cat Sager • Lindsey Simsik • Elisabeth Sinnott • Cora Skinner • Ellen Sloan • Eva Maria Smith • Erica Speights • Kaytlyn Spenner • Angela Sullivan • Laura Thomas • Paige Thomas • Kaitlyn Tower • Demi Trotter • Nancy Ukpe Gargula • Paulina Valencia • Ilona van der Ven • Jen Vu • Candace Walker • Charmie Warner • Jordan Younger

The 100+ women listed above were interviewed about their first year of motherhood. I am deeply grateful for their time, vulnerability, and the honesty with which they shared their stories. While no quotes or stories were used in this book, their words have profoundly shaped my understanding of this transformative year and the journey of matrescence.

Scan the QR code to stay connected

www.ingramcontent.com/pod-product-compliance
Lightning Source LLC
Chambersburg PA
CBHW030348130626
46549CB000C4B/1413